You Made It to Motherhood
A Guide for New Moms

You Made It to Motherhood
A Guide for New Moms

JENNIFER A. RODGERS

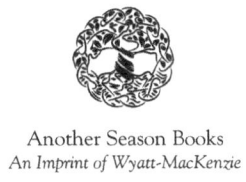

Another Season Books
An Imprint of Wyatt-MacKenzie

You Made It to Motherhood
A Guide for New Moms

Jennifer A. Rodgers

First Printing, 2018

ISBN: 978-1-948018-04-3

Library of Congress Control Number: 2017956608

© 2018 by Jennifer A. Rodgers

All rights reserved. This book or any portion thereof may not be reproduced or used in any manner whatsoever without the express written permission of the publisher except for the use of brief quotations in a book review.

Another Season Books
3320 Data Drive, Ste 350
Rancho Cordova, CA 95670

www.AnotherSeasonBooks.com
Visit the author's website at jenniferarodgers.com

To Haze and Jen – for your unwavering belief in me and constant support.

To Julie and Aaron – this book would not exist if not for the two of you.

Contents

PART ONE
Bringing Home Baby

1	A Major Life Change	1
2	How to Handle Change: A Growth Process	7
3	Your Growing Family: From Two to Three (or Four or More!)	15

PART TWO
Common Feelings and Realizations of a New Mom

4	Now You Are Her Mother, and You Are Much More Than a Caregiver	25
5	Strong Bonds: I'm Not Bonding with Baby (What Is Bonding?)	30
6	Feeling Guilty	34
7	Using Your Intuition	42
8	Yes, It Is This Hard—Don't Compare Yourself to Others	47
9	Deeper Struggles: Postpartum Depression and Anxiety	54

PART THREE
Coping Strategies for the New Mom

10	Time for You: Self-Care	73
11	Finding Support	79
12	Time for You and Your Partner	89
13	Sleep Deprivation and Trade-offs	94
14	Day-to-Day Life While Working or Staying Home: The Need for Routine	102
15	Views on Moms: We *Are* That Strong	109
16	Advice to New Moms and a Letter to New Dads	118
17	Full Questionnaires with Answers	125
	Recommended Reading & Listening	178

Introduction

My first thoughts and emotions after having my first child were ones of amazement, bewilderment, excitement, anxiety, happiness, and sadness, all mixed into one long night in the hospital. I could not believe that I finally had this baby that had been growing in me for forty long weeks (forty-one and a half, actually, and yes, that makes a difference to overdue pregnant women). I was relieved and overjoyed that we now had her to hold and touch, and yet I felt frightened and worried at the same time. *Now we have this baby, now what?* I thought. I did not know how to handle or cope with this new and monumental change. This is what we wanted, this is what we tried to achieve, and we did it: that was good, right?

Then reality sunk in. I have a human life to care for, what if she gets sick, what if she dies of SIDs, what if my husband dies from some horrible car accident and I am left to care for her all by myself? *How am I going to do this?* Suddenly, I felt scared and alone. As the weeks passed with our new little daughter at home, I began to understand just how hard motherhood is during this first year of life. I looked to books about motherhood and babies, but all I found were those that talked about how beautiful and amazing babies are, and how thankful we should be as mothers to have them, or humor books about the funny and gross moments. Where was the book about how our lives had changed by becoming new moms, how difficult this time is, and how to gracefully adjust to our new roles as mothers without judging or comparing ourselves to others? I couldn't find that book.

Thankfully, I found support through a new mothers' group at the local hospital. There I met women with the same fears, worries, and anxieties that I had. It told me that I was not alone. Almost all of the mothers there were having the same feelings as me. We shared our experiences and learned from each other. Still, once we left the group each Friday, we were on our own, searching, learning, and transitioning into this new role of being "a mom." As I witnessed all of us struggling on one level or another, I decided to write this book in hopes of helping every new mom transition more easily to her new life with her new baby. It was the book I needed and could not find.

This book is for all new mothers: those who already have their bundle of joy in their new nursery; those who are still waiting for that moment; and especially for those who are a little confused by the new responsibilities and changes in their lives. It is meant to help you through these times, to let you know that you are not alone and that other moms have been there, and to tell you that you *can* do this. Yes, it is hard; yes, it is challenging and frustrating and sometimes painful, but it is also miraculous and beautiful too. Slowly, we learn this as we share ourselves with our new little sons and daughters. Read this book for you, the new mother that you are or will soon be,

INTRODUCTION

not solely for your baby, or your partner, or society, but for you—because you deserve it.

Throughout this book you will read thoughts, feelings, views, and advice from other new mothers (these are italicized and in quotations) who have been through this transition into new motherhood. They attended the new mothers' group where I found help and reassurance. Their babies were all less than twenty months old at the time, so they remembered what it was like to go through the experience of a new baby in their lives. I hope all of our insights will be helpful.

PART ONE
Bringing Home Baby

≈ 1 ≈

A Major Life Change

"I think society really does not let the world know how hard it is to be a mom. We are all supposed to act like it is this wonderful thing all the time ... I don't think moms want people to know if they are not enjoying being a mom, because how dare you even think it? The truth is that it is a hard job, and society does not show that." -Nancy

I read the popular pregnancy books before I gave birth to my daughter. My husband and I took the classes on delivery (which I found scary instead of comforting). I went to the breastfeeding class. I talked to mothers with both young and older children. Few, if any, of these sources could prepare me for the life transformation that a baby actually brings. What was more frustrating was that no one warned me that this was a *complete* life change. Having babies and entering motherhood is so commonplace in our society that few people stop to think about how our lives are transformed by a baby. One reason for this might be that the women who have experienced motherhood, like grandmothers or mothers with grown children, quickly forget what it was like that first year. In the time span of your child's life there is so much that will happen, from his first steps across the living room floor to his stride across the stage at high school graduation, it is easy to forget what that first year was like. There are also those moms who blend into motherhood so easily that it appears they do not have the same experiences or feelings that many of us do. I am confident in my belief that these mothers are part of a very small minority, and even they have difficult times coping with the responsibilities of motherhood sometimes. There are some of us, too, who do not want to admit or accept this permanent change that happens in our lives. I wanted to have a baby, but I was afraid of the idea at the same time, and I did not want to believe that a baby would change me, my husband, or our marriage. My thoughts were: *What if this is not what I expect? What will happen? I cannot go back…right?*

For the majority of us, experiencing motherhood and a new baby is both amazing and shocking. Here is a human life that you and your partner made. She spent nearly ten months inside of you growing and developing, and here she is in your arms. The process of life is breathtaking and miraculous. It does not matter that humans and animals have been doing this for millions of years; when you are the one who has actively participated in the process, it is astounding. For the first few months of my daughter's life I marveled at the idea. I simply could not believe that 1) we created this baby who is here with us now, and 2) that she really came out of me! Right in front of me was a real baby who had swelled in my belly with her heart beating, her body moving around and showing up on the ultrasound. While I was pregnant I understood that she was there, but could not quite grasp it. Then, once she was out in the world, a tangible live human being, I was astonished. The change seemed to be instantaneous: one minute you are pregnant and the next you are a mom. I did not know what to make of it.

But, as we all soon learn with our babies' cries of hunger or discontent, they are here and they mean business. *Feed me, rock me, change me, hold me...wait, I don't know what I want!* my daughter seemed to say. And quite honestly, I had no idea what she wanted either. I felt like I was thrown into a play already in progress. I did not know my lines or where I supposed to stand on-stage. I did not even know what character I was playing. But everyone else did. I was "the new mom." And I felt like I was going to receive some bad reviews for my performance. I struggled to keep up with the needs of my new baby during the first few weeks. *Was she hungry? Did she have a dirty diaper? Was she hot or cold? Did she need to be swaddled or maybe have her blankets loosened?* Sometimes none of the answers applied. Sometimes it was just walking outside and seeing something new that calmed her down (or worked her back up into tears). There were no consistent answers, and I had a very hard time accepting that.

"I felt overwhelmed by the gravity of it [having a new baby]. I had never been in a role before that was a never-

ending, twenty-four hours a day, and that was entirely mine, even with my husband's support. I still feel there's never a real sense of utter relaxation, I mean in the way there was before I had another life to protect." -Kelley

I attended college and worked in an industry where there was almost always a right or a wrong way to do things. In school it is fairly straightforward: you perform the tasks asked of you and receive a grade for your effort. At work it is similar, you show up, do the duties of your job description, and receive a paycheck. It all makes sense. A new baby is quite different. We try to interpret what this little life needs when he may not know himself. The adjustment of just coming into the world must be overwhelming for a baby. He is nestled in a confined, warm, dark place listening to the steady sound of a heartbeat and other bodily noises. Then, probably without warning, muscles around him contract and he is pushed out into the world of bright lights, loud sounds, and a place that makes his body feel cold. Just learning what these new sensations are must be exhausting. (There is a reason we have no memory of our births, afterall; it is probably too traumatic for us.) So we care for him. We hold him, we love him, we offer him a breast or bottle, we try to make him as comfortable as possible in this new and strange world. But in the end, we really do not know what is going through his new and functioning mind. We do our best, but it might not be right. And if it isn't, then we often hear about it, *very loudly*. It is extremely frustrating to make blind guesses and not know whether it is the correct answer. Yes, the crying may stop, but does that mean the problem is fixed? Maybe, temporarily, *this* time. Grasping this understanding that the right solution doesn't always exist was extremely hard for me to take. *Why can't I plug in the correct number and get a solid answer?* Because, I realized after many months, this little being is human and she possesses the complexities that all of us have: emotions, feelings, needs, and wants. And she is just now learning what all of these things are, and who exactly I am, that person who holds her, feeds her, and tries to console her. Sometimes she might have been crying to release all those emotions that she did not understand. In the end, I felt just as confused as she probably did.

A therapist I know describes becoming a mother as a "growth process." We, as new mothers, are growing and changing almost as fast as our babies are as we accept this new role in our lives. The more we resist this change, the harder it becomes. It might seem unbelievable that you and your spouse were released from the hospital in charge of a brand-new baby, but you were. You are now parents. As we left the hospital, I sat in the backseat with our new daughter (yes, the paranoid new mom in the backseat) while my husband drove. It was a warm day for late October and the sun seemed especially bright. As we drove away, I cried. And cried, and cried. I blamed it on an influx of hormones and exhaustion. My husband looked nervously in the rearview mirror, "Uh…are you okay?" he asked. I assured him that I was fine, but the tears needed to come out. I suppose it was just a release after a very long labor, and the actual realization that this baby was coming home with us, ready or not. Our lives had changed.

"I was so worn out [after labor] I wasn't thinking much beyond 'get me out of this bed.' Then curiosity about the baby set in, followed closely by terror. I had never been around little kids before, let alone infants, and now I was responsible for this little thing?!" -Leisel

2

How to Handle Change: A Growth Process

"…For nine months I tried to prepare myself, but can you really ever prepare yourself? I kinda felt like I was still a kid and I still needed to be taken care of, and now I was responsible for someone else's life. I mean, was the hospital really going to let my husband and I leave with this baby…are we supposed to take a test or have a background check…are you sure we can take her? I am not so sure if we are qualified." -Nancy

These new changes are not all bad; they are just different. There are newfound joys in becoming a family. You three (or four or more) are a family now that can face life's challenges together, with you, mom, jointly at the helm with your partner or spouse (or solitarily, and this is okay too). However, with any change or transition in life, positive or negative, comes stress. If you are married, think back to your wedding day. Hopefully it was one of the happiest days of your life; now think of all the stress that went into planning that one day. Probably there were worries, fears, and concerns that this *one* important day wouldn't come out exactly as planned. And most likely it all worked out for the best either way. Even if it rained, you and your guests probably found a way to make it fun and special (memorable, if anything). Now think of this baby you might be holding in your arms right now, doesn't that wedding day seem easy? Or think back to moving out of your parents' house for the first time. It was probably exciting, scary, fun, and worrisome all at the same time. It took some adjustment and time to get accustomed to that new and different life, but you did, while learning quite a bit in the process. The same goes for having a baby. And, as you faced those challenges, learned, and succeeded, so you will in facing this change too.

First, you must accept that many parts of your life before the baby have taken a back seat for a while, and allow the new parts to make their way. Don't struggle to have your life be exactly as it was before your son or daughter came. This is a time of transition as you enter motherhood and become a mom. You are familiarizing yourself with this new role and letting go of many aspects of your "pre-baby" life. This was a hard time for me. Like most people, I am most comfortable with routine. My husband compares me to a cat: I am a creature of habit. I want to know what to expect as the day begins: get up, take a shower, eat breakfast, go to work, et cetera. A baby changes all of that. Suddenly, the biggest concerns are *when did she eat, is she hungry now, did she have a bowel movement yet, does she seem sleepy or gassy or lethargic*—the questions go on and on. Unfortunately, we are often so concerned with these details that we do not sit in our fancy glider rocking chairs, take a deep breath, hold our babies, and just relax knowing that, at this moment, everything is okay. Of course, we should always be concerned if there is truly something out of the ordinary or "not right" with our babies, but try not to overreact to every detail.

Doctors and pediatric appointments in the first weeks can contribute to these new worries and fears unintentionally. With our first child we saw a new and fairly inexperienced pediatrician who left both my husband and me scared and filled with anxiety as we walked out of our daughter's first doctor's appointment. Julie had lost half a pound and had not passed a bowel movement. The doctor sounded grave as he told us that she weighed less than her birth weight. He stressed that she needed to be gaining weight, not losing it. My husband and I fretted over this. I kept trying (and failing) to feed her when she did not want to eat, and my milk production was not keeping up (nor would it ever). We also agonized over her lack of poop!

The doctor made it sound like it could be near fatal if she did not start eliminating waste immediately. He suggested putting a thermometer in her rectum and taking her temperature because that can sometimes stimulate the urge to go. So we did. In the process I think we traumatized both her and us; and in the end, it did not work. We ended up seeing a different pediatrician three days later because the first doctor was not in our insurance group (another stressful fiasco, but it was for the best). The second, and very experienced, pediatrician had seen our daughter in the hospital after she was born, and had a much different take on the situation. We expressed our fears about weight loss and lack of a bowel movement. This doctor assured us that all of that is pretty typical. She said that most babies initially lose a little weight, due to the mother establishing milk production and the baby getting acquainted with breastfeeding. She also thought that Julie's first bowel movement would be coming soon, and not to stress so much about it. In her opinion, Julie's "issues" were pretty normal for a new baby. And, of course, the next day our daughter had the anxiously awaited poop (what a present for her parents!), and she began to gain weight as she should. All of that stress and worry over nothing! Granted, we were new parents, so the slightest "problem" seemed monumental to us, but looking back, if we would have taken a deep breath (and possibly got a second opinion), we could have saved ourselves much stress and anxiety instead of "praying for poop."

Since my husband had the opportunity to take a few weeks off of work after our baby was born, and I had the flexibility to have a few months off, we had no other distractions except to focus on our new baby and if she was doing the "right" things. If you are on maternity leave, or deciding to be a stay-at-home mom, just being at home all day right now probably seems strange too. Most likely you went to work or school and spent less than half of your day at home; now you are home all the time (in the beginning, anyway). Although home is a place of comfort, it also can be confining and isolating. Getting out of the house is refreshing and can be rejuvenating. Even if it is just a walk around the block, or a trip to the store (with baby in tow), it is nice to see the "outside world" again, because it is continuing even if you are not a part of it for a while (and that is okay).

I was so frightened to leave the house and go anywhere with our new baby. I do not remember what I was worried about exactly (probably, *what if she gets upset, what if she is suddenly really hungry, what if this is too much for her, what if she has a blow-out diaper*), so when my husband and I finally ventured out to a nearby little restaurant, I remember thinking that it was a major undertaking. You have to bring the diaper bag with every possible item you may or may not need: diapers, change of clothes (possibly two), wipes, bottle and formula (if not breastfeeding), cover-up (if you are breastfeeding), diaper cream, Tylenol, toys, you name it. Carrying a large and heavy bag around and remembering to keep it stocked is a chore in itself. Before baby you probably carried your purse (large or small) and that was it; now you have a new set of equipment for this tiny life. It is yet another little change that you are experiencing and that you might be struggling to accept. But soon you learn what you need to take, what can stay at home, or what to just keep in the trunk. It will all come in time, and eventually, your stress level will go down too.

"I always knew that I would be a mom, but I did not realize how much I would change as a person. The old me is a distant memory, and sometimes I still wish I still had a little bit of the old me." -Nancy

Not only has your outside world changed, but your body has too. Many of us gained weight with our pregnancies, some a little, others (like me) gained a lot. And your body does not lose all of that weight with the birth: you get rid of about 7–10 pounds of baby, and another 10–15 pounds of extra fluid, et cetera. The rest, we must accept, is our own body. After the birth of my daughter I went to the ob-gyn for a post-birth check-up. I asked the doctor if I had lost all of the weight that I would from the labor and birth, and if the rest of the weight was now a part of me. The doctor tried to tactfully imply that all of that extra weight was mine, and that I would not be losing any more due to the birth (thanks to my nightly bowl of ice cream, among other numerous treats). She said, "Uh, yes, those would be, um, fat cells." Fat cells! I had about thirty pounds of fat cells to lose, and I was dismayed. My life and my body did not feel the way I remembered them, and I was trying to understand and accept that I would not get them back in the near future.

I was told to not start exercising until eight weeks after the birth (due to stitches). I wanted to get started right at that moment, but I was told that, no, it was not recommended. Breastfeeding did not abate my appetite; instead, it continued to be ravenous at times. The pamphlets say that you burn off that extra weight with breastfeeding, but I did not believe it. How could I burn fat when I felt just as hungry to consume it? But after those eight weeks, I started to slowly work at those extra pounds; I walked and pushed that stroller (many miles) and changed my diet back to that of a non-pregnant person, and I eventually lost that weight. It is difficult and does not happen immediately, but if you continue to try, you will get out of those maternity clothes. Expect to continue to wear them in the beginning, however. And also know that you might have to donate those tiny jeans that were too tight before pregnancy, and that is okay.

Now, after having two babies, it is not surprising to me to see a new mom who looks a little overweight. In fact, one who did not have extra weight would be more alarming. After I had my second child I was very big all over (not just the belly). I gained more weight with my son than I did my daughter (I passed it off as the hungry boy making me eat all of the time). On the day of discharge from the hospital I went to the pharmacy to get a prescription and as I stood in line, there was a pregnant women behind me. An older man was in front of us and he said, "Well, isn't that nice, two women who are expecting." I was saddened that he thought I was pregnant too, but I did look like it, after all. I should have just smiled and nodded, but instead I told him (nicely) that I just had a baby and got out of the hospital an hour ago. He immediately reddened and apologized. I assured him that it was okay and told him that, after birth, women still have a lot of extra "stuff" to lose.

He apologized again and said that he had never married, he did not have children, and he just did not know all of that. "It is okay," I told him and I meant it. I was large, I'd just had a baby, and I had many pounds to lose.

A few would come off in the next few weeks, but I had many more to go—that was okay, that was a testament to giving birth. And though we might now sport some stretch marks, a C-section scar, or a few unwelcome veins on our legs, I say, be proud! You survived the amazing process of pregnancy and birth. You got through it like millions of other women, and that is something to celebrate. If this rite of passage means stretched-out skin, then so be it. We are strong and amazing mothers. Wear them with pride!

∽ 3 ∾

Your Growing Family:
From Two to Three (or Four or More!)

Having a baby completely changes "the way things used to be." Suddenly, your household of you and your partner includes one other person, a small one, yes, but the most needy one too. Now you are a family. Sure, the two of you might have dogs or cats, and considered yourselves a family before, with your animals as your surrogate children. But those furry little kids could be put outside when you did not feel like listening to them. You could leave the house and be assured that they would be waiting excitedly for your return. When we had our daughter, we had two dogs, two cats, and a turtle. I worried about how everyone would "handle" this new arrival. When we walked into the house with Julie in tow my husband set her down in her car seat on the floor so the curious animals would have a chance to "inspect" the new arrival. Almost all animals are simply interested and curious about new things, and letting them see and explore (gently) what you have will be much easier and less stressful on everyone than yelling "get away!" Our medium-sized dogs were not jumpers or overly excited, so I felt comfortable putting the baby (in her car seat) on the floor. The dogs sniffed her over and promptly lay down and took a nap. The turtle lived in a tank and could care less about what was happening beyond his glass walls. Our black cat looked down on my daughter from her cat perch, probably thinking, "Great, another human." But our orange cat, and my favorite, did not like this new little being. She looked at the baby then ran off, not wanting even to see the new (and loud) creature we brought home. When Julie would cry, Abbey (the cat) would howl right along with her. She refused to go anywhere near the new baby. She would come in the house and make a bee-line for our bedroom, her personal hideaway. Abbey used to sit on my lap in the evenings and purr. When I was pregnant she would use my big belly as a pillow. Now she voiced her dislike about this new change in our household. Having that cat skitter about anxiously and unhappily seemed to add to the difficulty of a new baby. "The cat doesn't even like her," I thought, "And she doesn't like me anymore because of this new change."

Slowly, though, Abbey came out of our bedroom. She would spend a little more time downstairs and give the baby a sniff or two. And, very, very slowly, she came back to her evening visits on my lap. Abbey, like most cats, did not deal well with the change. She rebelled against the crying and general disruption that our new family member caused. Although I did not want to admit it, I could understand her feelings. I did not want this new chaos in my life either. Having a baby was not at all like I pictured or planned. And I, like Abbey, did not respond well to the change either. I have learned over time that once I adjust to changes, after the transition, I feel confident and secure, but getting to that point is a challenge. A baby, as we know, is quite different from a pet, and in their first year, our lives are changed to suit theirs. The carefree days of going out to dinner or an afternoon movie have changed. Now arrangements must be made and planning ensued so that even the simplest of tasks become a challenge. However, if we recognize and accept it (and know that it is temporary), it really does help.

"I remember thinking, 'Wow, we're not watching her for somebody else, she is actually ours.' I also remember a moment when it really hit me that she was ALWAYS going to be there. It was no longer just the two of us. I was happy about it, but also a little scared and overwhelmed by it." -Teresa

But know that all of this change is okay because it unites you all as a family. As most of us have learned, family can be good and bad, but this family is yours. If it is just you and your baby, or you, your partner, and baby, you all form a unit together, a bond that can be made stronger and can support all of you. Initially, that was scary to me too, but it just took time to get accustomed to it, and I did. The first week out of the hospital, however, I was in a daze. My mother-in-law stayed with us to help out. She made dinner, which I did not feel like eating; she held the baby and rocked her; she cleaned the house; she ran to the store if we needed anything. I witnessed all of this in a fog. My daughter needed to eat every two hours and I struggled with breastfeeding. I had a hard time sleeping in between these short breaks, even though I was spent. I felt so out-of-sorts and discombobulated. On top of the mental fog I resided in, physically I felt poorly as well.

My labor was extremely long and exhausting (over ten hours), so my body was worn out. I had a sizeable tear from birth so I had stitches. I was constipated, as most women are after all of that, but was afraid to go to the bathroom due to the stitches. On top of it all, I got a yeast infection! All of the activity down there put my body out of balance so I was uncomfortable and itchy to boot. Needless to say, I was miserable. I called the doctor to see if I could use over-the-counter medication and the nursing assistant quickly told me, no, I should not put anything into the area in question, but just apply the cream around it, on the outside. I did that for three days and got no relief. At that point, if I was not already a wreck, I was on the brink. I repeatedly called the doctor for help, but I would either be put on-hold to leave a message (which went unanswered), or the line would just ring. I decided that I could not take this any longer. My mother-in-law, husband, new baby, and I loaded up in the car and drove the forty minutes to the ob-gyn. I went in, told the receptionist my problem, then sat down and waited to see someone. I told the poor lady behind the desk that I did not care how long it took, I needed to see someone *today*.

Looking at my sad, disheveled state must have had some effect on her because I saw the doctor soon after. She prescribed me a pill for the infection and it cleared up promptly. I could cross that problem off my list, at least. I also decided in that moment that if I had any more children I would not be using that doctor again, and I would get that pill before the problem became unbearable.

Eventually, things did get better physically. My stitches soon dissolved too, which helped, although the entire area was still extremely sore. Being so distracted by these bodily problems, in addition to the pressure of a new baby, I was thinking nothing about the joy of a new family; if anything, I was questioning what I did to put my husband and myself in this stressful predicament (blaming myself when it takes two to create a baby). It did take quite a while to accept this new family we created, but, like our Abbey cat, we slowly got accustomed to it and to the new member. As our new families get started with our babies we realize that we have broken away from our childhood family to form our own. It carries a lot of responsibility, but it is exciting and comforting too. Like everything else involved with this change, it takes time.

"Introducing a new permanent member to the family will bring changes. I think we work even better as a team now...just out of necessity. It also gives you a very strong mutual interest and love that transcends any hobby or other reasons you were brought together in the first place." -Kristen

Questions to Consider from Part One:

One of the most helpful things I learned to do for myself is to reflect upon my big experiences and write about them. Journaling helps me to clear away the buildup of emotions, feelings, fears, judgments, and whatever else is swirling around in my subconscious. I recommend reading through these questions and writing about them, but the choice is yours. Sometimes, just reading and thinking about them will be enough to help you make some realizations that you were not consciously aware of before. And those insights will help you process your experience, transition more easily into your new life, and help you to remember it better (because the first year of having your baby will drift away in a fog before you know it).

1) What were your ideas about having a baby before you had yours? Was it what you expected? Were you shocked or prepared for the experience? Write about your labor story and how you felt after first having and seeing your baby, and what you expected after bringing your baby home.

2) Do you ever feel confused or overwhelmed when you do not understand what your baby wants or needs? Is it different from trying to understand others' wants and needs? What do you usually do about it? Brainstorm some ideas.

3) Do you think that your life has changed dramatically post-pregnancy? How you feel about that? (Whatever you are feeling is okay.) How has your life changed? Write about your life now, how it is different, and how it makes you feel.

4) Has your body changed a lot (beyond the normal post-birth fluctuations)? Do you accept your body as it is or do you want it to change? Start writing your plan to get your body to a place that is comfortable for you.

5) How do you deal with change? Do you fear it, accept it, fight it, or "go with the flow" of it? Does it feel permanent? What are some of the positive and negative aspects of this change in your life? Make a list.

6) What does "family" mean to you? Do you feel like a family now that your baby is out in the world and part of your life? Write about how you feel about being a family and how you hope yours will be. Do you want it to be different from the family that you grew up with, or some aspects to be the same?

PART TWO
Common Feelings and Realizations of a New Mom

4

Now You Are Her Mother, and You Are Much More Than a Caregiver

"Yes, it is like your life changes overnight! One day you're pregnant and the next day you're responsible for a little life. It was hard to believe that I was really a mom." -Amy

During this time of our new family formation, I also questioned, *who am I now? I am now a mother. How did that happen?* Obviously, I knew how it happened, the process and the result. But what did it mean? I felt like I suddenly had gone from "married woman" to "pregnant woman" to "mother." The change seemed to occur so quickly that I was not sure what to make of it. Looking back, I realize that I was really seeking answers to the question, how do I cope with this change? I did not feel like a "mother" for quite a while after I had my daughter. The idea and role of "moms" in our society is so commonplace that those of us who become the "mom" do not get the chance to understand what it means, to feel out the territory, and to process the new responsibility that we are now in charge of someone's life. In our society the ideal "mom" does it all, knows it all, has everything organized, and is in control all of the time (and still has energy for her spouse in the evening). That is the way it often is portrayed in television commercials, but those ads do us a great injustice by creating standards that are unrealistic and unattainable. We are moms and we are human.

We also incorporate the role of a mom from our own mothers. Regardless of whether your mom was ideal or not, that version is your experience and it is instilled in you. Depending on how you look at it, making the comparison of your own mother to the one you want to be can be good or bad. If you had a loving, wonderful, supportive mother growing up, you might strive to be like her. However, if you didn't and you came out with many negative experiences, you might try too hard to be nothing like her. We often try to make up for what we believe are our parents' shortcomings by doing the opposite. Instead of trying too hard to be like your own mom or not like her, just be the best version of you that you can be. Your baby will be more than happy with that.

> *"I remember the first day I really felt like a mom. She was just a few days old and I had been up with her all night. I was listening to a lullaby CD with her and it hit me that I was a mom and that was something I had always wanted to do. I was amazed at that point how much she meant to me! It was a great moment!"* -Amy

Amy's moment is indeed special and intimate. It is also a moment that we all expect to have because of the image of the gentle and giving mother that we hope to be. I did not feel like this mother, and I was sure that there was something wrong with me because of it. I felt like a caregiver (and a milk machine) instead a mother. *Anyone could fill in for me and my daughter would not know the difference*, I thought. Is this true? That is debatable, but the more you take part in your role as mom: changing, feeding, rocking, talking, playing with your child, the more he will come to see that you are one of the most important and stable forces in his life. It may not be the way you planned or thought, but the more "grunt work" you do, the more your baby will see you as the person to rely upon and trust; and, in that process, create a healthy attachment to you. That said, your partner should also be involved. Any man who says "I don't do diapers" does not realize that even this unappealing task is a chance to connect with your little one—to make eye contact, to hear a soothing voice, to be a consistent person in your baby's life—and that is extremely important for both parent and child, whether you are the child's birth parents or not.

"I would say after the birth [I felt like a mom]. Meeting her needs, soothing her, and giving her love and comfort all made me feel like her mom." -Teresa

Teresa's comment above shows that it really does come down to how you look at a situation. I did not feel like a mom while I did all of the tasks a new infant demands. I was exhausted and confused, and worried that I was not "doing it right." Yet if I looked at it from Teresa's point of view, I might have adjusted to this new role of mother a little quicker. Remember that you are an essential figure in your baby's life. It might feel like you are merely "Chief Diaper Changer" or "Midnight Feeder Extraordinaire," but you are much more than that.

"I tease my husband that I feel like 'The Keeper of the Baby,' not her mommy." -Renée

It is a different experience for every woman when the role of "mom" is accepted and feels true. Looking back, I probably resisted that too. Since I had so many expectations that I did not meet, I did not realize or know at the time that it was all okay and that it would just take time. My moment of truly feeling like a mom came when my daughter just turned two. We were in a restaurant with other family members and my aunt said, "Who's that?" pointing to me. My daughter said, "Mama!" and I was stunned. *She really knows who I am*, I thought. More than likely, she had known it all along; it was me that needed the time to let it settle and acknowledge it. Once I did, however, I was really proud to be Julie's mom.

"I think I started feeling like a mother in the first few weeks when I became the expert on this little person. I knew her routine, and what she needed when, better than anyone else. I

was the only one who could provide certain things for her, and that made me feel like she was mine." -Christina

5

Strong Bonds:
I'm Not Bonding with the Baby (What Is Bonding?)

In the birthing classes the teachers often recommend that your newborn infant be placed on your bare chest immediately after birth. This will ensure an immediate bond, they say. Whether or not this is true is not my place to say, but this happened to neither of my children after birth. My first baby, who took quite a long time to get out into the world, was blue and not breathing. The first order of business was the respiratory therapist to get the poor thing breathing air. As I mentioned earlier, I had a sizeable perineal tear that needed to be mended, so that delayed holding the baby as well. On top of it all, I was so exhausted from such a long labor that I remember crying and feeling glad that the process was finished. I told the nurse to let my husband hold the baby first because I was so tired that I thought she just might fall out of my arms.

I did hold my baby soon after my husband did when she was breathing regularly, wrapped up in a little pink cocoon, and somewhat placid after everything that she experienced. At that point I was more amazed and dumbfounded that she was finally here than in the throes of bonding with my daughter. In the following weeks I still did not feel "bonded to the baby." I was not sure exactly what that meant. I struggled to keep up with her daily needs; so relaxing and simply rocking her did not bring on the feelings of attachment that I thought were necessary, or so I was told. When I asked other moms, "did you immediately bond with your baby or did it take a little time?" only three out of eleven felt that they bonded with their babies right away. The rest of the mothers felt that it took time.

"It took a while [to bond with my baby]. My daughter was very fussy and cried more than most babies (from what I've been told). It was hard to develop that bond when I was sleep-deprived, impatient, emotional, and completely overwhelmed. I'd say it took a few weeks." -Renée

"It took me some time to really bond. My daughter had jaundice and was put back into the hospital to be treated. Then by week two she still had jaundice because I did not produce enough milk. She was a very fussy baby and it took us a good month to figure each other out. I feel horrible saying that because now I totally bond with her and have this indescribable love for her." -Nancy

"It took a little time. I would say about a month or so. It was really hard at first because I was in a lot of pain. I had a third-degree tear along with having trouble with breastfeeding. I think it really hindered bonding right away. I knew I loved her, but the bonding took some time." -Amy

All of the special importance that the medical and "baby community" put on bonding might make us wonder, what exactly *is* bonding with my baby? Bonding is often described as the attachment you feel to your baby. To me it is what makes you be right by his side when he cries, or what makes you know you could suddenly have superhuman strength if someone attempted to hurt him. I think of it as somewhat primal. It is something that all animals possess: that need to protect and defend if necessary (in the days of animal predators). And it is something that is there all along, even if you do not feel it immediately. If your baby needs medical care and is in the hospital (like Nancy's experience), there is not much you can do except be present when you are allowed. But most importantly, do not put more pressure on yourself if you do not feel an immediate bond. As you continue to care for your baby, most likely you will start feel closer and more connected to him (if you are still very worried that you are not, see the section on Postpartum Depression and Anxiety). As you learn how he likes to be held, what he does when he is hungry or full, and as you change that mountain of diapers, you are bonding with your baby. Kristen says it best below.

PART TWO: *Common Feelings and Realizations*

> *"I feel bonding with your baby is a process. He is like a kindred spirit that you have known for a little while, but that you have never seen before. And this new person in your life is very needy and demands all of your time and energy. The love is always there, but it takes a while to recognize the parts of you and your husband wrapped in this new body."* -Kristen

Like adjusting to the changes of having a baby and bringing him home, bonding can take time. Letting it happen naturally is the best course to take. Fretting that you do not feel what you think you *should* be feeling will only add more stress and make you feel guilty, which no new mom needs. And that leads us to the next topic...

6

Feeling Guilty

"...Motherhood is such a full-time job, from breastfeeding every few hours, to changing, maintaining sleep schedules...I've never been an ultra-scheduled person so I found it difficult to curb my ability to go for a run, dash to the store, or meet up with friends around a baby schedule. I tried, and I felt guilty whenever she fussed, because I wanted to push the jogger a little farther or find one more thing at the store." -Kelley

As amazing as motherhood can be, and as much joy as it can be to cradle your little one in your arms, unfortunately, what also often comes with this new role is a host of guilty feelings. From not breastfeeding to letting him cry for few minutes to not having the latest gadgets or for just needing a break, there are so many reasons that we new moms can feel like we are blameworthy. We are doing this to ourselves, in the end. We are choosing to feel these feelings of guilt, *but* it is also very difficult to not feel them sometimes.

PART TWO: *Common Feelings and Realizations*

> *"I probably feel guilty on a daily basis. Do I hold her too much or not enough? Am I loving her enough...does she know how much I love her...is it okay for her to cry, do I entertain her enough? All of these questions go through my mind on a daily basis."* -Nancy

My biggest reason for feeling guilty in the first few weeks of motherhood was because I wanted to give up on breastfeeding. I was having a terrible time trying to do it and my body did not seem to produce what my baby demanded. I really wanted to quit, but the guilt of it all kept me trying, and trying, and trying. As the posters and pamphlets in the ob-gyn's office tell us, breast milk is the *best* diet for a newborn (and until they are twelve months old, or so they say at the moment). We are told about the benefits of it for our babies; we are told that it will help us new mothers get rid of some of that pregnancy weight; and we are told that formula just does not cut it for your new baby. And you want to do the very best for your new baby, right? Yes! That was the answer resounding in my head, but the reality of it all was quite different. I was not prepared for the pain and difficulty of breastfeeding, the art of getting the baby to "latch on," the uncomfortable feeling of having two very full boobs that leaked while I slept and sometimes for no apparent reason, making me carry an extra shirt in the diaper bag.

In the hospital the lactation specialists would come around occasionally and see me struggling. They would maneuver my daughter into a position, grab a breast, tickle the baby's face with it, then shove it forcefully into her mouth. I sat there, mouth open, wondering if that is really what I needed to do. Julie would slowly begin to nurse with a vise grip on my nipple. I would express this pain to the nurse who would tell me that I was doing it wrong and would then take Julie off, squeeze my breast, and shove the entire thing into the baby's mouth. The pain continued anyhow, but I let the nurse do it all the same. Soon it would be over and we would do it again forty-five minutes later. It did not take much time for my nipples to be raw and blistered. They hurt to the touch. Still, feeling guilty for denying my daughter food literally from my breast, I continued this painful process. Often she would not "latch" and I would try over and over again while she cried and tried to eat and I fumbled. I felt terrible.

After we went home, without the lactation specialists there to guide me, I continued to attempt to feed her from the breast. She wanted to eat every two hours so my husband would get up, bring her to me in the middle of the night, and I would try again. I was exhausted and in so much pain, but I felt too horrible and shameful to stop doing it. We went back to the hospital and I paid a lactation specialist $75 for an hour of her time to help me get it right. She told me that my milk production was low and that I should pump to increase it. She also performed the same act that the other lactation specialists did and that I somehow could not do correctly, but I continued to try and imitate it. At home I unearthed the breast pump that I got from the baby shower and got it working, attempting to do the specialist's recommendation.

Still, even with the pump and its mechanical endless drone, my breasts were only producing so much milk. In the middle of the night I sat at the kitchen table, dead tired and shirtless, while the pump droned on. *This is one of the saddest moments of my life*, I thought to myself. I felt worthless because I was an inefficient milk machine that could not generate enough product. When I finally got two ounces out and no more would come, I turned it off and gave up. We put it in a bottle and gave it to Julie. She did not drink much of it; apparently, this time she was not hungry. In the end my mother-in-law ended up throwing it out. I sat there, stunned, "You—you threw it out?" I asked incredulously. "Well, it had been sitting there awhile, so I figured that it wasn't any good," she replied. "Do you know how long it took me to get that?!" I wanted to scream at her. But I didn't. Instead, I cried and thought more about this breastfeeding situation because I did not know what to do; however, what I was doing now was not working.

I felt like a failure. I watched other women do it, without any problem, it seemed. In the new moms' group one of the moms remarked how she was *determined* to breastfeed her baby. She said that she was going to figure it out, whatever the cost. *What was wrong with me*, I questioned. Maybe if I just try harder, I reasoned. So I did, and it still was not getting any easier, only more painful and wearisome. I ended up talking to my cousin's wife about it. My cousin called from the East Coast to congratulate us on our new baby and he put his wife on the phone. This was a person I had met maybe three times and didn't know well, but we were now fellow moms. So when she asked me how I was doing, at my wits' end, I told her about my hard time with breastfeeding. I was in near tears as I spilled out my pain and frustration. She told me simply to stop. I was stunned. "Stop what? Stop breastfeeding? But what about all the nutrients and the benefits, and the things that everyone says about breastfeeding your baby?" I questioned her. "Don't let those boob Nazis get you down," she said, and told me that my baby had received my milk and gotten the antibodies from it already. She also said that I should not feel bad about it; lots of people she knew had needed to stop breastfeeding for various reasons and their babies were fine.

I thought about this possibility. *Should I stop? Is that an option I can take without feeling horribly guilty?* My husband had already mentioned the idea, but I dismissed it. I was the mom here; I was the one who was supposed to be capable of doing it all, not him. But after talking with my cousin's wife, I thought, *maybe she is right. Maybe I can stop and the world will not condemn me.* So I did. We bought formula and our daughter took it just fine. My husband and I took turns at night getting up and feeding her. I was not woken up every two hours to try to feed a baby without enough milk to give her. Dividing the duty and having enough food to offer helped me immensely. Although I wished I could easily whip a breast out and comfort my

PART TWO: Common Feelings and Realizations

baby like other moms, I was glad that I could still feed my baby and could see that she was thriving all the same.

"Sometimes I do [feel bad], especially when it comes to the fact that I didn't get to nurse her for very long. I sometimes feel guilty about that. I try to remind myself of how difficult it was and that hopefully for the next baby I will be more prepared for the challenges. Also, I try to remind myself that I did the best I could." -Amy

This is *not* a push to get you to stop breastfeeding. I repeat: *I am not endorsing mothers to stop breastfeeding.* This story and the quote above is meant to show you that you do not have to feel guilty about not doing the absolute best thing for your baby. You need to take care of yourself as well. That was the right decision for me in that moment. It also eased my guilt about not being able to produce enough milk (yet another fruitless guilty feeling!). The point here is that we new moms have enough to deal with just adjusting to this new life with our babies. We do not need to add guilt on top of it. Give yourself a break in general, whether it be feeling guilty about letting yourself take a long shower or buying the off-brand of diapers. As long as you are doing your best, you have no reason to feel guilty—so don't.

"Sometimes I feel bad when she cries and I lose my patience with her. I try to learn from my mistakes and do a better job the next time around." -Teresa

Alleviate Feeling Guilty: Watch out for "Shoulds"

A "should" is anything that you think you "must" do or "have to" do, or else something negative will result (often, by being judged by others or yourself). "Shoulds" can be hiding in all sorts of situations and we just don't realize we're thinking in such a way; all the while, they are causing us to have feelings that rarely benefit us. For instance, "I should write those thank-you notes for the baby's presents," "I should call my aunt back and find a time for her to see the baby," "I should clean the house before my in-laws come over." Usually these "shoulds" are not things that absolutely need to be done. On the contrary, they are things that we feel we have to do because of guilt or fear. The sooner that we can recognize and drop them, the better we will feel.

Using the example, "I should write those thank-you notes." Most of us agree that thank-you notes are polite signs of gratitude, but do you really need to send them? Will anyone refuse to speak to you again if you don't? We fear what others might think of us if we don't send them, so they turn into a "should," and continue to weigh on you until you do it. The next one, "I should call my aunt back," involves both guilt and fear. You might feel guilty if you don't find the time for her to see the baby; she is rather lonely and it would make her feel good to see a new baby. Plus, if you don't call her back, she might get upset at you and you don't think you can handle any family drama at the moment, so you give in to the "should" and make the call, not because you want to, but because of the hypothetical outcomes if you don't. The last example, "I should clean the house," is another should that is ruled by the fear of what the in-laws might think of you if they show up and find a messy house where their new grandson now lives. What will they think of me, you might wonder. More than likely, they will understand that you just had a baby and have quite a lot happening at the moment. A messy house is not your priority right now, but our worried sense of self doesn't see anything rationally.

The best way to think about these "shoulds" is to question if they answer a "need to" or "want to" in your life. Go back to the first example with the thank-you notes. Ask yourself, do I need to write thank-you notes?   No, you don't. The world will not end and people will not die if thank-you notes are not received. So, then ask, do I want to write thank-you notes? You might genuinely enjoy writing thank-you notes and connecting with people, so if that is the case, then yes, go ahead with the plan of writing them. It might give you a little down-time and the chance to reflect on people's generosity. But, if you're too tired and really do not want to write them, then don't, and leave it at that. Stop the wondering and pondering about what people might think and let it go, because most people are very understanding, or they won't notice that a thank-you note didn't show up. If you still really have a problem with it, then schedule the task on your calendar six months from now when things settle down. You just had a baby, people will understand.

The next one, "I should call my aunt," use these same two questions. Do you need to call your aunt? No. Again, nothing terrible will happen if you don't call. Next, do you want to call your aunt? Maybe you really like your aunt and find her to be a comforting presence and you do want her around, so call her. But, if your answer is no, you don't want to call her because she is emotionally-draining or you find it is more work for you when she is around, then heed your feelings and don't call. She is an adult and will survive.

The last example, cleaning your house for your in-laws. Do you need to clean your house for them? Definitely not. Do you want to clean your house for them? It would be hard for me to say yes to wanting to clean my house after having a baby, but who knows, maybe you really enjoy the process of cleaning. Or, maybe you can meet yourself halfway and agree to a general pick-up and straighten, but forgo the vacuuming and dusting. That way you feel a little better about the state of your house, but you are not sacrificing all of your time and energy to a full cleaning.

Try to stop and notice when a "should" comes up for you. The best way to find them is take a moment and make a list. Start with anything, "I should..." then fill-in whatever pops into your head. "I should start using cloth diapers," "I should put on make-up before I leave the house," and let them keep coming. You might find that you have a very long list. In that case, start going through each one and asking yourself if it is a "need" or "want." If it is neither, just cross it off the list; you don't need them hanging around and making you feel guilty (just the act of crossing them off can help). If you find that your list only contains a few, try to notice your thoughts over the next few days, sometimes these shoulds aren't so obvious. When you do uncover one, write it down. As you continue to notice them, ask yourself if they are a "need to" or a "want to." You will find that you can clear out many unnecessary thoughts and feelings of guilt or fear by going through your "shoulds," which will help you immensely in the end. As someone aptly put, "Stop should-ing on yourself!"

7

Using Your Intuition

"I had more support than I needed. I learned quickly to nod politely and say 'thank you.' Then do whatever I felt was right. Following my own instincts was always the right path."
-Renée

We have all heard the phrase "a mother's intuition," and most of us probably dismissed it as nothing more than a common saying, but even if you believe in it or not, you should always "go with your gut" or "follow your heart" (whichever phrase rings true to you). It means just stopping for a moment and letting yourself feel and know what you think is the right thing to do as it pertains to your baby and her care. We all have this ability—mothers and fathers, women and men. Our culture seems to emphasize it more in the view of the mother, possibly because women are often allowed to express their emotions and let that hidden side surface (men are often supposed to be "logical and rational" despite what their gut might be telling them). So if you are burdened with endless questions like, "Should

I feed her now or wait?," "Do I hold him or wait a minute and see if he stops fussing?," "Does she seem ill enough to take to the doctor, or will they think I'm the paranoid new mom?," just stop for a minute, take a deep breath, try to clear your mind, and see what your gut or your heart says. You might realize that he will be okay if he talks to himself while he lies in his bassinet for a minute longer and you finish dressing, or that you are truly concerned about your baby's health and the doctor's office can think whatever they like, you want to know that your baby is okay.

If I had stopped listening to other people (individuals and books included) and simply did what felt right, I could have saved myself so much stress and anxiety. But I did not trust myself. I did not want to make a mistake and be blamed for it. As a result, my baby and I probably suffered from all of that worry and anxiety. Just like the section on guilt, give yourself a break and trust yourself. What do *you* think is the right thing to do? Let your true feelings tell you, and do not put so much pressure on yourself or your partner. Parenthood is new to all of us, even those with older children; we are all still learning each day with each new age and stage of development. No one does it perfectly; and those who say they know the absolute correct way to do it should be questioned. You know your baby best, even if you are still getting to know each other. You and your partner are the people who determine her care and are responsible for her, not the books, the experts, or the latest fad. And you have it in you to know what is best for your baby.

"...when you read the how-to-deal-with-your-new-baby books, take the advice with a grain of salt. I remember treating the suggestions as gospel and feeling like a failure when it didn't work. You really have to trust yourself and remember that your child will be okay. I can't count the number of times in the beginning I would sweat small things, like the fact that she wasn't on a fixed schedule or she was small for her age. The truth was, genetics and her personality played a bigger role in those things than I did." -Teresa

When my second baby came along, I was already familiar with the process of having an infant—the feedings, the midnight diaper changes, the "fussy" time during the day, so I thought I was pretty prepared, but he was a completely different being than my daughter. After Julie reached a certain age, we could put her down in her crib at night, following the ritual of books and a bottle, and she would drift off to sleep on her own. Some nights she had trouble, as all of us do occasionally, but for the most part she got herself to sleep by herself.

My son was very different. He needed someone with him while he fell asleep. He took comfort in knowing that someone was beside his crib and that he was not alone. This was initially very difficult for his dad and me. We were used to putting the baby down and that was that; now we could have a little break. We were frustrated that he could not just "go to sleep." If I followed some of the books available at the time, I would have let him "cry it out" for as long as he needed, then after three magic nights, he would do it on his own. This did not work for us. I attempted the "cry it out" method for one night and the poor boy was so beside himself with screams and tears (which still did not end after a very long period of time) that I knew this was not the right way for him. He simply wanted someone near him to feel safe and comfortable while he went to sleep. My intuition and my gut told me that having him scream and cry to sleep until he finally succumbed to exhaustion was not what he needed. So, we stayed with him at bedtime after the books and bottle, with the lights turned down low. One of us would stand by his crib and let him know that we were there and that he was okay. Was it what I expected after the first child? No. Was it easy? No, especially when my husband was working late and I struggled to keep my toddler waiting quietly outside of the room while Aaron went to sleep, since he would have stayed awake if she were there (even though she claimed she could be very "quiet" in his room, I quickly learned that she couldn't).

But I knew that this was the right way for us. I wanted him to feel safe and secure, so this was what he needed. If I were to put the question out there for the experts to answer I probably would be told by one side that I needed to get over it and let him cry, that both he and I need to "toughen up." And on the other side I would have heard that I should be lying down with him, he needed me and the closeness, and that we should have been co-sleeping from day one. What I settled on was what he responded to and what I thought was right. In the end, you and your partner are living with your new baby, not the experts. They are not getting up in the middle of the night to change him, you are. If what you read or hear makes sense, then definitely incorporate it into your parenting, but if it does not, then just let it go. Seeing how often methods and theories change, it tells us that there is no definite "right way," because inevitably it will change again in a few years. Knowing that, the choices should be made by you, not them.

"Nobody is perfect. Not me. Not you. Not your mother. And not your mother-in-law, no matter what she says! You can only do what you think is best and make the decisions that work best for your family. Again, follow your instincts." - Renée

8

Yes, It Is This Hard:
Don't Compare Yourself (or Your Baby) to Others

"Hardest job ever." -Kelley

One of the most surprising, and possibly disappointing, aspects of being a new mom is realizing and accepting that this job is actually really hard. You just do not fully understand that before you give birth, not until you are fully responsible for a life, twenty-four hours a day, seven days a week. Even when you get away for a short time, you are still thinking or worrying about that baby. It is a lot of pressure. As I mentioned in the introduction, I tried to prepare myself for this new role, but there really is no way to do that until your baby is in your arms. It is like trying to read and learn about swimming: only once you are in the water and actually doing it do you fully understand what it is like, and the only way to truly learn. We can have certain expectations of what the water will feel like, we can watch and predict the task to be easy or hard, or that we might love it or hate it just by watching other people do it and knowing ourselves. However, our expectations are just ideas that we create in our heads; they are often not the reality of the situation. I majored in English in college. I enjoy literature and occasionally get to read it aloud, especially very old works like Shakespeare. I had a vision before I had a baby that during those midnight feedings I could softly read literature to her while I fed her then rocked her back to sleep. "Ha!" I thought to myself once I was finally there at midnight, fumbling in the near darkness to change her diaper (because no one wanted bright lights at that hour), and closing my eyes while I fed her and rocked her because I was so tired that it hurt to keep them open. The mere thought of Shakespeare at that hour would have made *me* cry. But, as a mom-to-be, I did not know what I would be facing; and that is okay, that is how we learn.

"I thought being a mommy would be so fun, and always wanted kids. I also thought that pregnancy would be pretty easy and that newborns would just sleep all the time (ha ha!)"
-Amy

As both Amy and I learned, our expectations of having a baby were very different from the reality we faced once we had our babies in our lives. We must try not to be too disappointed when reality does not meet up to our expectations. After all, they are just stories we create and want to believe. If the life you have with your baby is not what you expected, that is okay. The majority of us moms thought it would be different too, but do not let that bring you down or take away from the joys you can experience as a new mother. You may be tired and not ready for another night of feedings, but the look of wonder your baby sometimes gives you in these moment is still something to be savored. It is hard, yes, but try to get the most out of the little payoffs.

"I have a new-found respect for my mom, as well as any mother that I see out and about. It is the hardest job, but the most rewarding job. The day your child smiles at you it makes all the difference, and nothing else really seems to matter."
-Nancy

Mothers are everywhere, in every country, across the world and throughout history. They too were once new moms. They also experienced what it was like to finally hold that baby and to feel the exhaustion that goes along with caretaking. But that is hardly ever addressed, at least not often, and especially not in the United States. People do not look sympathetically at you in the grocery store or on the airplane while you struggle with a crying baby; they look annoyed, at least most do. Fellow moms typically have been in that same position, so they might give you an understanding glance, some a warm smile. Why we keep this secret about the hardship of new motherhood is something that I do not understand. Maybe, as our babies turn into young children and then we have another baby, and as that baby turns into a child, we forget how hard it really was during that first year. Those painful memories fade into the distance as we address the current issues of our children in the moment. But it is helpful to know that you are not alone; most women have been in your position and got through it just fine. And, it is also comforting to know that there are many women in your same place at this same moment throughout your city, the country, and the world.

"I used to think mothers all had it together. Many of them make it look so easy. I think this is why I was so depressed early on, because I did not have it together and was nothing like what society portrays a mom to be. Now, however, I realize how unrealistic society is." -Tanya

Sometimes just acknowledging that yes, it is this hard, can help. If you are thinking, "Wow, I did not expect it to be this tough. Am I the only one who feels like this?" No, you are not. And also know that if you see a new mom who seems completely put together, handling this new role like it is second nature, acting as though her life has not dramatically changed after this new addition, she is fooling you. We all deal with and handle change differently, but no one can claim to be completely unaffected after having a baby, including adopting one. And it does not help you in any way to compare yourself to that mom anyhow. Her experience is different from yours. She is

PART TWO: *Common Feelings and Realizations*

going through her own set of challenges, rest assured. Smile at her, even if she does not smile back, and know that you share a special experience with her.

One of worst places to start comparing yourself is by looking at pictures of "friends" on social media and thinking that your life should be like theirs. For whatever reason, we try to paint a perfect picture through our postings: "Look, he's three months and smiling!" or "Wow, she's crawling in a princess dress, how cute!" You never see the postings with distraught moms like, "Oh my God, if I get spit up on one more time, I'm going to scream!" or "Please make him stop crying, please, what do I need to do?" No one wants to admit their pain or vulnerability when showing themselves to the world, and I am not saying they necessarily should in all situations, but just don't go down the path of "compare and despair," because you will not come out feeling good about yourself or your life with your new baby. Connect with others, share special moments if you want to, but put the screen down before you realize that you think you "should" be like other moms.

"I seem to spot moms around I think are pretty close [to being perfect]…or are they? My husband tries to remind me there's always a side you don't see." -Kelley

A friend of mine recently had a baby and she seemed to be adapting to the "motherhood experience" fairly well. She looked tired, but did not seem overwhelmed, and her family commented on how much she was "enjoying the baby." I immediately compared myself to her and told my husband that I did not handle having the first baby so easily. My husband, being the nice and supportive person that he is, started to tell me that her situation and circumstances were different from ours. Then, probably with the prompting from him, I realized that my experience was *my* journey and I cannot compare it to others. Her experience is *her* journey, and it has nothing to do with me, just as mine has nothing to do with hers.

When we compare the details of our experiences, our reactions, and thoughts, then feel bad about it, we do no service to ourselves. I was meant to have the somewhat traumatic, but very instructive experience of having a baby and learning to accept how my world changed because of that. My friend was meant to have a different experience, and the two experiences cannot be compared or judged; they just are. Every person is unique, and so every experience is unique as well. We share this experience of having babies, and possibly our stories could be similar, but they are not the same. Instead of feeling shame or anger that I "should have" handled my situation differently, I decided to accept that our journeys were very different, but we still can honor each other by what we share.

> *"Sometimes I feel guilty for being competitive as a mother—like wanting my kid to reach milestones before others. What's that all about? It's very silly. All kids develop at their own rates and the great majority turn out just fine!"* - Christina

One of my favorite sayings is "This too shall pass" and it will; whatever situation you are in, it will change. The only constant that we can depend on in life is the changing of it. After I had Julie and I was in the midst of my breast-feeding struggles, beyond exhausted, and feeling nearly crazy, I spoke to a good friend on the phone who lived on the other side of the state, but thankfully, we still kept in touch. As she asked about the baby and how I was doing, I struggled to keep back my tears. She recently had a baby too, who was less than a year old, so she understood my situation at that moment—a new mom with a newborn.

I told her how I was so tired and that Julie was not getting enough milk, that I was feeling terrible, anxious, and depressed. She told me that she understood this time is very difficult, but it does not last long. She said that it was only a few months in comparison to the years that we would have her as a child. I could not see that. I was so stuck in that moment of pain and exhaustion that a few months felt like a few years. I could not comprehend that this difficult time would pass and that one day I would feel better again. It did not seem possible. But she was right. Time did pass, my daughter did sleep through the night eventually, I started feeling like myself again, and life continued to change again. And it will for you too.

"My view of motherhood has totally changed. It is the toughest and most important job in our world. I have so much new wonder and respect for my own mom, having raised two children. I don't know how other moms can make it seem so effortless, knowing how tough it really is." -Kristen

9

Deeper Struggles:
Postpartum Depression and Anxiety

"I was completely overwhelmed and underprepared. I remember crying on my bed telling my husband that I just could not do this. I suffered from depression after my baby was born and had medical issues related to an emergency C-section. I thought I would never be able to be the mom I wanted to be."
-Tanya

This is a subject that is very close to me because I experienced postpartum depression and anxiety with both of my children (anxiety is sometimes listed as a symptom of the depression, but I think it can stand alone and that a mother can suffer from mostly postpartum anxiety and less depression, though often the two go together). Please note that I am not a medical doctor, or claim to be an expert in any medical field. I am only sharing my personal story in hopes that it will help other moms who might be having similar difficulties after having their babies.

PART TWO: *Common Feelings and Realizations*

After you give birth, your body is undergoing many changes hormonally. It is trying to equilibrate back to its non-pregnant state. As a result, many women experience a range of emotions from elation to depression; but this tumultuous time is not supposed to last too long (some say roughly four to nine days after birth), and is commonly called "baby blues." When symptoms continue then it is time to start thinking about the possibility of postpartum depression or anxiety. Many women experience baby blues; one statistic estimates up to 50 percent of women (according to the Illinois Department of Health). It is a much smaller percentage for those who have postpartum depression or anxiety: about one in nine women (according to the

After delivery: What is happening in your body?

After the birth of your baby your body immediately begins to change hormonally. The hormones that were sustained during pregnancy drop quickly (mainly estrogen and progesterone), and your body starts to recalibrate to its non-pregnant state (excluding the hormones needed for milk production). As a result, you might feel a whole range of emotions throughout the first few days after you give birth. You might feel elated one moment then teary the next, then angry, then happy again. Think about how you were while pregnant or if you often suffer from PMS, then multiply that by ten. After the birth of my second child I remember feeling very awake and not physically tired until the third day. My hormones were helping me to stay awake and react if my baby needed me. Once that third day passed, however, I was exhausted and needed to help my body recover. So if you feel like your emotions are continually changing, that is normal. Just take a deep breath and know that they will soon settle. If it feels like nothing is changing after the first few weeks and you are still feeling unsettled, overly sad, or depressed, have the courage to talk to your doctor about it.

Centers for Disease Control and Prevention). Those who have been through a time of depression or anxiety previously in their lives are at a higher risk.

Part of the difficulty for me during this time (which lasted mainly from birth until about the time my daughter was one year old), was that I was unclear about my symptoms and had trouble determining if my symptoms meant that I truly had postpartum depression (PPD). Then, if I was experiencing it, and once I admitted that to myself, what would I do about it?

As I described earlier, the birth of my daughter was very long and difficult. It left me beyond exhausted and with many stitches (from a sizeable tear). I could not sleep well in the hospital with all of the activity constantly happening, and I found it painful to just sit down and use the bathroom! So even upon leaving the hospital I did not feel prepared physically for the new changes that would happen at home.

My mother-in-law stayed with us to help out with the new baby, as I mentioned earlier, and my husband and I were both grateful that she was there. It felt like she was the only one who had any experience with having an infant in the house (and she was). As I tried to breastfeed my daughter, and was continually woken up to have her nurse again, my exhaustion only grew. I did not feel like I could sleep soundly, and I knew that sleep was what my body and brain needed. That pressure only made matters more difficult. Everyone kept saying to "sleep when the baby sleeps," but I could not do that so easily. I have never been a person who could sleep anywhere or at any time. I was accustomed to darkness, quiet, and a relaxed environment in which to hopefully drift off. Now it would be two in the afternoon and I would drag myself upstairs to fall on my bed and hope that sleep would come. It often did not.

As this unusual sleep/wake cycle continued, the fog that I felt surrounded by only grew thicker. I was in a constant daze and out of touch with the world. Television, often a good distraction, was just noise that I could not focus on. And when my husband would put it on a show that I used to like, such as a *Friends* rerun, I only felt more distant from these people who lived carefree lives in New York City. Were they getting up with a baby? Did they have any major responsibilities? I could not relate to any of it any more. Soon it reached a point that when the sun started to set I would feel incredibly anxious. A feeling of dread would start within me at the thought of another hard night, rushing to sleep while the baby slept, and jumping at every noise thinking that she was waking up again.

When I went to the ob-gyn for my follow-up appointment after birth, the doctor asked me how I was doing. I told her that I was having a very difficult time sleeping and that I could not seem to stay asleep or go to sleep when the baby slept. She looked at me with very sympathetic eyes, but said that she did not know why that was happening. I asked her if there was anything I could do or if this was normal, and she shrugged, not having an answer.

I left feeling hopeless and confused. I did not fit into the typical postpartum depression symptoms; at least, I thought I didn't. Looking back, I obviously was feeling many of the symptoms of depression and anxiety at that time, including sleep problems, which can be common with depression (and yet even the doctor did not recognize it).

Crying became a common occurrence for me. There did not need to be a reason for my tears; they just came. I could not understand why I was feeling this way or what I could do about it. My mother-in-law stayed for a couple of weeks and did her best to help us. She cooked and cleaned and loved holding her new granddaughter. She made us lasagna one night and for once I was very excited. I still felt so hungry while I was breastfeeding. My body needed that extra energy. But as she put the plate in front of me and I smelled the delicious scent of carbs, cheese, and tomato sauce, I suddenly had no appetite. It was so strange. I wanted to eat; I was hungry, and it seemed so delicious just a moment before, but now it did not seem appetizing in the slightest. I felt like I could not touch it. I ate a few bites then left it. Today I know that this episode was also a symptom of the depression I was feeling, but at that time I could not understand it. I never had an experience like that before, so I was confused and did not know what was happening to me or why.

My mother-in-law went back home and my husband had to go back to work a couple of weeks later. We were lucky that he was able to take some time off to be with his new daughter, and now it was up to me, "the mom," who

PART TWO: *Common Feelings and Realizations*

was in charge of caring for this baby. I was so scared. I did not think I could do it all on my own. We live in a rural area and the isolation of that frightened me. It was just the baby and me for at least ten hours a day. The "what if" possibilities I came up with kept me paralyzed: *What if she gets sick and I can't get to the doctor; what if I end up sick and can't care for her; what if something happens and I can't handle it?* It would go on and on. But, despite my fears, I stayed home day after day with my baby. In the end she was fine. She did what normal infants do: sleep, eat, poop, cry, look around, gurgle, and coo.

I was not fine, however. I could take care of my daughter, but I felt very alone and I cried often. One day while riding in the car with my husband and the baby I was crying—again. My husband did not understand what was wrong with me and what he could do to help. Through my tears I told him that I woke up and waited for him all day to come home so that I could go back to bed again, only to do it over the next day. He did not know what to say. He felt just as helpless as I did as he watched his wife falling apart.

Even though all of these symptoms are so obvious to me now, at the time I was alone and miserable, and not wanting to be a new mother with "postpartum issues." It felt shameful. I felt flawed that something was "wrong with me." I was able to hide it well. While at the mom's support group I attended I did my best to seem like I was doing okay, not great, but surviving fairly well, like the rest of them. When I did get up the courage to talk about my sleeping problems and what I could do about it, one mom, who was a nurse, told me that I would be put on an anti-depressant and that I definitely did not want to do that. She was very against any medication or any other substance that was not completely natural for herself or her baby. I took those words to heart. I did not want medication anyhow; that would be admitting that I had postpartum problems and that I needed to be medicated because of them. So instead, I suffered, as did my husband, and my baby to an extent. As time passed the pain and the feelings of despair and sadness dissipated, but it took a very long time. I saw a therapist, and talking through some of my feelings did help, but my daughter was well over one year old by the time I felt like "me" again. My sleeping continued to be an issue and my doctor prescribed me something to take when I was really having a difficult time, and it helped, but I tried not to take it often.

By the time my son came along, nearly three years later, I could look back at that time and understand that I should have sought help, regardless of whatever shame I felt. The feelings of pain were still memorable and I was worried that I might experience them again. One week after being home from the hospital with my second baby those same feelings came back. I was not as teary as I was with my daughter, but that same anxiety and despair crept back into my life. I knew these feelings by now. I knew they were a part of postpartum for me, so I made an appointment with my ob-gyn (a different one than the first time), and told him that I was having feelings of depression and anxiety, that I had them with my first baby, and that I thought he should prescribe me something for it. He understood and we talked about the different medications he could prescribe. He suggested an anti-depressant, and this time I agreed. He explained that being on an anti-depressant would help with the feelings I was having, but would not solve my problems. He said that it would not make me feel happy all of the time or out of touch with reality. Although I was scared to start the medication, I knew that it was the right decision for me in that moment. I did not want to suffer through that again; I also did not want my family to either. I now had a newborn and a toddler; I wanted to feel my best and to be present for them and my husband.

After being on the anti-depressant for a few weeks I did notice a difference. That heavy feeling of dread, the anxiousness at seeing the sun go down, and the overwhelming need to cry over anything went away. Life was not perfect, of course: having a baby and a two and a half year old is extremely challenging, and there were times when all three of us were crying at once, but it was an episode that passed. I felt like myself and I knew I could get through this difficult time of infancy and lack of sleep. I knew that my hormones would go back to their pre-pregnancy state and that I would be okay. I am not advocating medication for everyone; that is a personal choice, but for me it was the right one. It was not easy for me to start it, and it was also difficult to stop it after that year had passed, but I am glad that I made the decision to take it. It helped me, and my family.

Postpartum depression or anxiety is still a "hush-hush" topic for women, but it clearly exists and should not bring shame. Out of twelve women from the new mom's group, myself included, three of us admitted to having problems after the birth of our babies. That would equate to one in four women having some type of issue with PPD or anxiety. So, how can we help ourselves with this taboo topic? It is very difficult to talk about having these problems even when we are not currently feeling bad, and once we are in the middle of it, it becomes even harder. I openly discuss my experience now, but at the time I was afraid. I did not want to be judged or admit that I was feeling so terribly. In our society babies are meant to cuddled and enjoyed with moms in some type of love hypnosis where they do not feel depressed or any negative emotion. This is very unrealistic and it is to our detriment.

The first step in dealing with postpartum mental health is to arm yourself with information. Following are a set of common symptoms for PPD and anxiety. Most women experience multiple symptoms. If you do not think you fit with these symptoms, but still feel very badly or not like yourself, you could be suffering. Write down anything you are feeling and see how long it lasts. The period of "baby blues" is not supposed to last longer than a week or so after the birth, so if more than a few weeks have gone by and you still do not feel right, start to think about the possibility of postpartum depression or anxiety. Remember, it does not mean you are flawed or unable to be the best mom, it just means that your body and brain are having a harder time adjusting to this new change in your life and establishing the equilibrium they had before pregnancy and birth. You are still a good person and will be a wonderful mother. Recognizing and doing something about your mental health is the bravest step to take; it can be scary, but you are not alone and *will* feel better again.

Common Symptoms of Postpartum Depression

(If you have only one symptom, it does not necessarily mean you are experiencing postpartum depression.)

If you are feeling:

- Extreme sadness. You cry a lot, even when there is no real reason to cry.

- Overwhelmed.

- Guilty, because you think you should be handling motherhood better than this.

- Irritated or angry. Having little patience or being annoyed by everything.

- Like you are not bonded to your baby.

- Very scared or confused.

- Empty or numb, like you are just going through the motions.

- Hopeless, like nothing will change or get better.

- Like you are a failure, or weak and unworthy; or feeling disconnected from the rest of the world.

- You are having trouble sleeping. You cannot get to sleep or stay asleep; you cannot sleep while the baby sleeps. Or you sleep constantly, without the energy to get out of bed. This goes beyond the mixed-up sleep schedule a baby brings.

- Having trouble eating, having no appetite; or you cannot stop eating because it seems to make you feel better.

- Having trouble concentrating or focusing. You have trouble making decisions and your brain always feels "foggy."

- Having disturbing thoughts that you cannot control.

Common Symptoms of Postpartum Anxiety

(If you have only one symptom, it does not necessarily mean you are experiencing postpartum anxiety. Also review the symptoms of PPD; they can be intertwined.)

- Racing thoughts. You cannot quiet your mind or relax.

- Excessive worrying. Having lots of "what if" thoughts: "What if the baby doesn't wake up, what if I can't handle this, what if I can't get to sleep?" You are afraid to be alone with the baby because of all of these worries.

- You are busy all the time and cannot settle down. Instead of resting you are cleaning the house or doing more laundry; you feel like you must constantly be "doing" something or have the need to leave.

- Having disturbing thoughts that you cannot control.

- You feel constantly anxious or on edge.

- You having feelings of dread or that something bad will happen.

- You have no appetite and do not want to eat. You feel nauseous.

- Physically, your stomach is jumpy or in knots; you have headaches or just do not feel "right."

- You may feel the need to check things constantly. Did I lock the door? Did I lock the car? Did I turn off the oven? Is the baby breathing?

- Having trouble sleeping. You cannot get to sleep or stay asleep. You cannot sleep while the baby sleeps.

- You feel like nothing will change. This is your life now, and you will always feel this way. You feel hopeless.

Help for Postpartum Depression or Anxiety

Although it might feel like you are all alone in this journey, know that you are not. Help is available and you *can* start to feel better. The hardest and biggest step is realizing and accepting that you might have a problem in this area. If you have made it that far, congratulations, you are braver than you think. I sought out my doctor the second time I felt the weight of depression and anxiety, after the birth of my second child. I recognized the feelings and knew that I would continue to feel badly unless I sought help. If you are unsure, do a little research and see what other mothers have gone through. Thankfully, the Internet is full of websites now where women are unafraid to share their stories. One excellent site is **www.postpartumprogress.com**. They have stories, symptoms, resources, and help for mothers. I wish this site had existed while I was in the midst of my postpartum depression. I was afraid and ashamed, but it is easy to be anonymous on the Internet and find information without giving away your identity.

Medication was the best route for me at the time, but that is not the only way to feel better during this dark time. You might have reservations about taking medication, or you are nursing and worry about the effects on your baby. This is understandable, and the decision is solely up to you. Try not to feel pressured into thinking that medication is the only path to feeling better, because it is not. Talking with a therapist or a trusted friend can help. I met with a therapist for a short time after my daughter's first birthday. I was feeling more like myself, but still was not one hundred percent "better." Speaking with someone who is trained to understand difficult feelings and issues was very helpful to me. She was that neutral party who could assure me that I was okay and remind me that this is just a short period of time in my life, as well as helping me deal with issues at that moment such as being a new mom and how that affected my marriage (which also changes considerably after a baby). Self-care and support (see chapters 10 & 11) are also big components to helping you feel better. We often hear about the example of the mother and child on the airplane and the mother needing to put on her air mask first, then her child's, if the plane is in a state of emergency. This is so true. If we cannot take care of ourselves then we cannot adequately care for anyone else. Cognitive behavioral therapy (CBT) is also beneficial. This is a fancy term for recognizing your defeating thoughts and replacing them with realistic and positive ones.

Depression and anxiety after the birth of your baby can be a long road, but it will go away over time. It is hard to see or accept that in the midst of your pain, however. People who have never experienced this type of depression or anxiety cannot fully understand what you are feeling. Seeking help can make that long road so much shorter and less rocky. Do it for yourself and your family.

Questions to Consider from Part Two:

One of the most helpful things I learned to do for myself is to reflect upon my big experiences and write about them. Journaling helps me to clear away the buildup of emotions, feelings, fears, judgments, and whatever else is swirling around in my subconscious. I recommend reading through these questions and writing about them, but the choice is yours. Sometimes, just reading and thinking about them will be enough to help you make some realizations that you were not consciously aware of before. And those insights will help you process your experience, transition more easily into your new life, and help you to remember it better (because the first year of having your baby will drift away in a fog before you know it).

1) Did you feel like a mother after having your baby? Do you feel like one now? Describe why or why not.

2) Do you ever feel like you aren't the "ideal" mom? Why? Is it due to unrealistic expectations of yourself, comparing yourself to others, or an unrealistic image in your mind? Can you identify any expectations of yourself that you think you are not living up to?

3) Was there a special moment when you realized and accepted that you are someone's mom? Describe the experience. If it hasn't happened yet, that is okay!

PART TWO: *Common Feelings and Realizations*

4) Did you feel bonded to your baby right away or did it take a while? What does bonding mean to you?

5) When do you feel guilty, as it pertains to your baby? Are these feelings warranted or are you being hard on yourself? If a friend told you the same reasons for feeling guilty, would you think that she should feel that way?

6) Make a list of your "shoulds" in regards to your mothering or to your life in general. Go through the list and see which are items you "need to do," "want to do," or are neither. Cross those items off the list that do not fulfill a need or a want.

7) Have there been any times when your intuition (or gut) caused you to make a decision, or a time when you didn't listen to it? What was the outcome?

8) What were your expectations about being a mother before you had your baby? Were they very different from the ways things are now? Is that disappointing to you, or are you okay with that?

9) Did you think motherhood would be hard? Were you surprised by the answer?

10) Did you experience a range of emotions after giving birth and bringing your baby home? What were they? Do you think you experienced "baby blues"?

11) Have you experienced any symptoms of postpartum depression or postpartum anxiety? What are some ways of helping yourself during this time? Make a list. If telling your doctor about the way you feel is too scary, why? What are your fears? Sometimes writing them out and looking at them critically makes them less scary.

PART THREE
Coping Strategies for the New Mom

～ 10 ～

Time for You:
Self-Care

"After seven years of marriage and career, it was a challenge for me to give up the simple things I liked to do for myself, like reading magazines. Free time just vanished, and I don't know if anything could have really prepared me for the reality of that." -Christina

Christina's quote is so true: your free time does disappear once a baby enters the picture. When we were pregnant women and reached that nine-month mark, we wanted that baby to come out so badly. We were uncomfortable physically, tired of sleeping on our backs and struggling to bend over, and we were excited to meet this new little being. However, once he does enter the world, it's "go time," so to speak. After that, we, as mothers, rarely get a break. And that is why it is so important to make sure you get some time to yourself and to do it for yourself. You have entered into a twenty-four hour a day, seven day a week job that does not stop. If that were a job in the working world, the government would require that you take breaks every two hours, but we moms do not give ourselves those mandatory rests. And yet, both our babies and ourselves benefit from having short times away from each other. This does not mean you pack up and leave for the weekend (unless you feel ready to), but it does mean that you go out and get a cup of coffee (or decaf herbal tea, whichever you prefer) with a friend and without baby. You start reading a brain-candy novel that will get you hooked. You watch a television show (by yourself) that will take you to a different world or listen to your favorite podcast or music. Your baby is not going anywhere, and will be happy to see you when you return (even if he cries a bit when first seeing you, it is okay, you still deserve and need time to yourself).

"[If I could do things differently I would have]... researched out more things and tried to give myself a little more 'me' time. I really neglected myself and my needs, and I think it affected our lives a lot." -Amy

Unfortunately, for many of us, it is only in hindsight that we realize that we should have allowed more time for ourselves. I had an unrealistic idea that since I was "the mom," I was the one who needed to be with my baby all of the time: I needed to comfort her when she cried, I needed to get up during the night, I needed to prepare her bottle—all me, all of the time. And I would feel very guilty when I finally broke down and needed to take a break. This was not beneficial to me or my baby. On Mother's Day when Julie was seven months old I decided that I earned that day and I was going to get a pedicure. I did and I enjoyed it thoroughly; and when I got back home after my day away, I felt so much better. I felt like I had more patience. I was excited to see my baby and my husband. It gave me the chance to miss them. Being around Julie all of the time never gave me the opportunity to see how she was around other people and to let me feel like my life existed beyond motherhood. Even if you go back to work, full time or part time, you still need time for yourself. Work is work; it is not you choosing what you want to do with your time. Although work can be a good distraction, it is not the same as treating yourself and appreciating that moment.

Cathy Adams, an author and partner in the podcast Zen Parenting Radio, calls these short breaks "mini-freedoms." It is giving yourself a small amount of time that is entirely for you. Your spouse or a family member will probably need to help you give yourself these mini-freedoms by watching the baby and allowing you to have this free time, but it is more than worth it. My uncle told me that when his wife started having babies, he would be sure to give her a little time to herself each day. He would take their baby for a half hour or an hour and let his wife read a book or rest or do whatever she felt like. He realized how important it was for her to have a little "me time" after being with their baby all day. I wish I would have heeded his advice because I know my husband would have supported me, but I did not. Instead, I felt completely overwhelmed most of the time. You still can, however. So find a way to have some "mini-freedoms." If you really cannot find someone to help out, then take the opportunity at nap times. Instead of cleaning house, doing mountains of laundry, or planning dinner, take a few minutes just for you. Start this habit: you will be glad that you did.

There is one important aspect of this advice that you already are learning now that your baby is here (or will be soon), which is that you will not be able to finish any task completely in one sitting, and that is how it will be for a long time to come. I can tell you that the sooner you accept this, the less frustrating the experience will be. It took me so long to acknowledge this fact because I was simply not used to being constantly interrupted while I tried to do something (thus, why it has taken me so long to finish this book). For instance, your baby is finally napping and you decide to pay some bills instead of reading a book because they will not pay themselves. As you sit down with your checkbook and pile of mail or your computer and start to organize things, the baby starts to cry, you go to the baby's room, soothe him, he gets quiet, you leave, and go back to your piles of mail and bills. After you remember where you were and figure out how you were organizing everything, the baby fusses again, so you go back to the room, do the same thing all over again, and come back to the same piles with the same questions about how you were organizing them. This may happen at least three more times, and you may even reach the point of opening your checkbook or computer and staring blankly at it, until he cries again and you reach the point where you want to abandon the whole bill-paying idea and just sit in the baby's room because he obviously is not napping this afternoon. Yes, it is extremely frustrating, and you might remember those days of getting out the checkbook, balancing it all, then even filing those paid bills. Unfortunately, I can tell you that such a task will probably take you twice the time it used to, but instead of getting angry and rallying against it, just accept it. We all know how difficult it is and understand the frustration, but it will not be this way forever.

I attempted to get back to exercising after the allotted "no strenuous activity" time passed when my son was a few months old. That thirty-minute routine took at least an hour between me stopping it, running upstairs, soothing him, coming back down, pressing play, exercising for about three to eight minutes, stopping it, running upstairs…you know the rest. And although I was very frustrated that I could not just do my short bout of exercising and get rid of all those extra pounds already, I reasoned that I probably burned more calories by just running up and down the stairs a dozen times. So, if you can, try to find the positive in all of it because it will take quite a few years before you will be able to complete a task without at least a few interruptions. If anything, just laugh at the craziness of it all.

"I'm at home five days a week. I'm amazed by how much I can get done during a two-hour nap, and yet how little I seem to get done at the same time." -Kelley

11

Finding Support

"I had the support of my husband and family; however, my family lives out of town and my husband works very long hours. By day three, I was left alone to figure out this baby and Mom stuff. I had to figure it out and by week two I went to Mommy and Me because I needed support and I thought I was possibly going crazy." -Nancy

As I mentioned in the introduction, I found a huge amount of support attending a new mothers' group at our local hospital. Initially, when I saw the flyer in the packet from the hospital I thought, "Well, that's nice for some new moms, but I think I'll be fine." Boy, was I wrong! After battling exhaustion, postpartum hormones, depression and anxiety, as well as doubting myself and my abilities to be a mother, all the while wondering if our lives would ever be "normal" again, a weekly support group was a tremendous help to me. Although the shy introvert in me wanted to continue to hide at home, I made myself go (at least once, I reasoned). I found mothers there with infants and babies ranging from a couple of weeks old to nine or ten months. The room was big and open, with the tables and chairs all pushed to the side. The moms would come in, lay their blankets and babies down, sit cross-legged in a big circle, and openly discuss any topic that someone brought up. The unspoken rule of the group was that once your baby started to crawl, your time at the group had ended. No one needed a newly crawling baby excitedly and unknowingly mowing down newborns and creating disaster in his wake. All of the moms understood this and abided by the rule.

The facilitator was a very caring and compassionate mom whose kids were grown. She sympathetically listened to us new mothers struggle with issues of breastfeeding, co-sleeping, colic, or any other problem, and would help us think up solutions while reassuring us about our ability to be moms. She understood, more than we did, that our babies were not the only ones growing, we were too. I met new moms there who, just like me, questioned themselves on the "right" thing to do, and who wanted to be the best for their babies. I felt relieved just knowing that other brand-new moms existed out there; it helped me to realize that I was not alone in this journey.

"We have no family in-state, so when my mom's visit after the birth ended, we were on our own. I remember feeling quite isolated. It was nice when I started attending the new moms' support group. Meeting women going through the same struggles and joys helped." -Teresa

PART THREE: Coping Strategies

I attended the group with my daughter from the time she was four weeks until she was nine months old (when she started to crawl). It was with sadness when I stopped going. Everyone there was helpful and supportive, and it gave me confidence in my abilities as a new mom. I looked for a similar group for older babies, but could not find one. I even tried to start one myself, but did not get many responses in our small country town. It seemed like all of the activities were for toddlers starting at age two. I really missed attending the group and connecting with these other moms. We lived about forty minutes from the town where the hospital is located, so it was a trek to go there. Some moms would get together for play dates at nearby parks, but it was always difficult for me to make those meet-ups work, given the distance and time it took to get there. My baby would no longer just go to sleep for the ride. She wanted to be out of that car seat instead of sitting backwards and staring at the rear window of the car. I felt very isolated after leaving the moms' group; and years one to two with my daughter were hard. I did not realize how important it was to have people around to help or just listen to my latest "baby issue."

"I went to a new moms' group, which was invaluable in providing a support network. It was like a big brainstorming session on everything from gas to diaper rash to marital relationships. I would encourage any new mom to seek out a group. It was good to get out and talk with other people who actually wanted to hear me talk about baby stuff. I also had a lot of help from friends and people in my church." -Christina

Connecting with others helps to relieve the overwhelming weight of these new responsibilities and why support is so important; however, it does not have to come solely from a support group. Local family or friends can be helpful; neighbors or people in your church (if you attend one) can also be a source of support. If you do not have anyone nearby, a phone call is a substitute, but at least it is a way to reach out to other people. When Julie was still a young baby, she would have a "witching hour." It was typically around 4:00 or 5:00 in the afternoon or early evening, and during this time she was extremely fussy. Nothing really seemed to help except holding her and walking. In our house we could walk in a small loop from the living room through the kitchen and back again. I walked that loop over and over again, day after day, during the witching hour. If Julie became calm and placid, I would set her down, only to have her wail the moment she felt her back against the crib, so I would pick her back up and walk, and walk.

Sometimes during this "walking hour" I would telephone my best friend who lived across the country, or other people I had not spoken to since the arrival of the baby and my extrication from society. My daughter did not mind me talking; we just had to keep moving. I learned that I did not have to walk around in circles feeling helpless or resentful; I could catch up with friends or relatives and still comfort my daughter at the same time. This was pre-Facebook, Instagram, or any other social networking site. Now lots of new moms share their lives with their Facebook friends and probably feel a connection that they would otherwise not have. I think it is another way to find support if you do not have anyone nearby. Just be sure not to spend your life doing it! Your baby is growing up before your eyes; try not watch it happen via the latest post, when he is right there in front of you waiting for you to interact with him.

"Don't be afraid to ask for help, because it's surprising how much friends and family will want to help but just don't want to interfere." -Kelley

Sometimes the hardest part with getting support is letting people help. It can be difficult to ask for support, and admit that you need it, but we all do, regardless of how much someone appears to have it all together. Looking back, I would have asked for more help, from friends or relatives. My mother-in-law and my aunt were available certain days of the week and very helpful, but I could have asked others. I just did not feel comfortable doing it. My own mother lived three hours away so she was not an option, but I had co-workers who would have loved to have a baby for a few hours. If you are worried about letting someone else care for your baby, start out small by leaving for an hour or a quick run to the store. The person whom you trust with your baby is most likely competent enough to handle everything for a short time. One person I worked with offered to come over and just clean my house. I turned her down. Why?! Someone is willing to clean my house, *for free*, and I did not feel right accepting her help. Today, I would tell her to come on over!

"I feel guilty all the time. It is hard convincing myself it is okay to get a babysitter and go out. I deserve some down-time. My child deserves a break from me now and then too. Having a break makes both of us appreciate each other more and strengthens my relationship with my husband. You read that it takes a village to raise a child. I believe that completely... sometimes you have to look hard to find your 'village,' but find it and let them help. It was also hard for me to convince myself that when people offered help I should take it—it was not an imposition on them... they OFFERED!" -Leisel

Your biggest support, however, is the person who you spend the most time with beyond your baby—your spouse or partner. The two of you are in this together. Even if society seems to place most of the responsibility on the mother, the fact is that you both are intricately involved in raising your child, and you are both responsible for the life you jointly created. When my husband would stay home with our daughter while I was having some time away and someone would ask him if he was "babysitting" that night, my aunt would always point out, "No, he is parenting, not babysitting. It's his baby too!" And that is true; our child is half of him and half of me. So it makes sense that your spouse should share in the duties involved with his baby. Even if you stay at home and he works, he can still do his share. If you and the father are no longer together, he still has a responsibility to the baby that he helped to make.

The problem comes when we mothers do not let our partners do anything. Either from fear of him making a mistake or from thinking that, as moms, it is solely our job to take care of the baby. The latter was my own mistaken belief: *I am the mother, so it should be me dealing with the baby all the time, twenty-four hours a day.* Again, who can do a job day and night endlessly without ever getting a break? No one! We all need a rest, and hopefully your partner is aware of that. More than likely, he will not take that into consideration unless you point it out and have a conversation about it. I am not saying that he will do this on purpose and try to shirk his responsibilities, but if you continue down the path of doing it all, all the time, without a word to the contrary, then why should he change? To him his life will be more or less the same, except that his wife is really tired and now there is another person to add to his health insurance. When that scenario happens, the person who is doing all of the work (i.e., the mom) typically gets angry and resentful.

"In the beginning it definitely changed my marriage negatively. My life had totally changed and my husband seemed to continue as business as usual. I really disliked him for that. I didn't feel like he knew what I was going through or like he was even helping me. I clearly had the baby blues and had no clue what I was supposed to do. I was the one getting up in the middle of the night to feed while he slept next to me, snoring."
-Nancy

Save yourself and your marriage from experiencing a very difficult period by sitting down with your partner and having a conversation about the baby and all of the duties involved. Let him know that you both are in this together and that you need some help. I remember being upset because my husband did not know where the acetaminophen was in our house if the baby had a fever and needed some while I was not there. To me it felt like he was not caring or pulling his weight with the baby if he did not know how to get her medicine, should she need it. But instead of sitting there and stewing about it, I should have just had a conversation about it: "Let me show you where I put the medicine and thermometer in case you need it." It could have been that simple, and eventually it was, but I took his ignorance as a sign of his lack of caring, which was something I created in my own head, and not necessarily how he truly felt.

Instead of going down that path of mistaken beliefs and ideas, get it out now so you are both aware of each other's feelings. Your views on parenting styles might be different as well; have the discussion now. Do not wait until you are both exhausted, the baby is wailing away, and you are arguing over whether she should cry it out. In those stressful moments we usually lose our cool, say things we do not mean, and end up feeling resentful or regretful.

"I think we're striving for a common goal more now and we do agree on parenting skills, which is huge. The most difficult part is a bit of resentment I have for my husband's freedom.

He still meets up with friends for lunch, drops by the store or hair salon after work, etc...tasks that for me require an act of Congress. He is very involved and supportive, but I feel he'll never understand the full-time nature of motherhood. I think he does manage to relax in a way I never quite accomplish."
-Kelley

  As I said earlier, I mistakenly took on the belief that the baby was solely my job, and it took quite awhile for both my husband and me to realize that we needed to work together. We both enjoy working outside or working on our house, and always have a list of projects going. After the baby came along, my husband would continue his weekend projects and I would be "stuck with the baby." He would go about his day thinking about his to-do list while I sat there feeling angry and bitter. I did not think to stop him and say, "Okay, now it's my turn to work on something; your turn with the baby" because in my head, the baby was all my job. After we worked things out, my husband was more than willing to do his share, and more than happy to give me a break.

  I see moms all the time taking on all of the responsibilities and thinking their husbands are incompetent or unwilling before even giving the guy a chance or having a discussion about dividing responsibilities. I can tell you that if you decide to have a second child, it only gets harder. I am not trying to dissuade anyone or put a negative spin on it; I only say this because, if you do not let your husband help or talk to him about it now, once you have that second baby, you will have double the work to do. You will have a newborn and another child, and you will be trying to manage both (think about how hard just one is!). As you watch your partner doing whatever he wants, you will be considerably more upset and angry that he is not helping as the newborn cries and the other child has a tantrum because the baby is crying. So, sit down and talk about it now; it is worth it.

"I got very mad at my husband for a while too because he was going on with life as usual and I had to do 'baby duty.' His life wasn't seeming to change at all, while mine got turned completely upside down. I resented that a lot. Eventually we figured out we needed to talk about the changes and our feelings and we worked through them, but it was rough for a while."
-Leisel

～ 12 ～

Time for You and Your Partner

"Yes, having a child definitely changed our marriage. When she was born, we had just celebrated our one-year wedding anniversary. So we were newlyweds and also just had a baby. We spent a lot less time together and it really strained our marriage in the first year. What I learned is that while a new baby changes so much, it's important not to neglect the relationship. Ours is getting much better now (our little girl is almost two), but it was definitely affected it in the beginning." -Amy

Another aspect of motherhood that I did not want to face initially was that having babies will change a marriage. I liked my marriage and my spouse as they were; I did not want anything to change that. We were happy and we wanted to stay that way. But, the reality is that any big and permanent change in a relationship will affect it, at least in the beginning, until those ripples of change can settle and the people in the relationship adapt. (Change, good or bad, creates stress; and stress affects any relationship.) In this case, you and your partner created a life, literally, a living human being. Without the two of you, that new little human would not exist. You are both responsible for that, which is somewhat scary, but amazing too. The point is that you both have invested in something major, a part of you and your partner exists together in this little baby.

You have a connection now that you did not have before, and it is wonderful to share it together, but let us go back to a time before this connection existed, before pregnancy and discussions of names and the anticipation of the coming of this little one. Way back when (or so it feels like) when it was just the two of you enjoying each other and your company together. What did you like to do together? Go to the movies, enjoy a nice dinner at a new restaurant, go bowling, rock-climbing, scuba diving? Remember what that was and take time to do those things with your spouse, if possible. We all know that you cannot drop everything and go scuba diving, but you can have an afternoon or evening out where you discuss where you want to scuba dive some day (and you will, really), or look at pictures from a previous trip, reliving fun memories together.

This can be a hard task: just like finding someone to look after the baby while you have some "me time," it can be difficult to find someone so that you and your partner can have some "us time," but really try to carve out some time for just the two of you. One mom in the moms' group I attended said that she and her husband had a "date afternoon," by having pizza at Costco then going for a walk afterward. That might not be the most romantic experience, but it is valuable time for you as a couple, doing something together, minus baby.

"I was very surprised at the difficulties having a baby brought to my marriage. All of a sudden I felt my husband and I were strangers." -Tanya

If you and your partner are feeling like Tanya, then it is crucial to have some time together and get to know each other again. You might be seeing a different side of the person you thought you knew so well, and he might be seeing a new side of you too. You are a mother now and most likely would do anything to protect your baby. Your husband might be taking a back seat for a while as you adjust to these new feelings. However, when you combine that with the exhaustion, stress, and the enormous weight of responsibility that you both feel for this little life, you might look at your husband, or he might look at you, and think, "Who are you?" You both might need to work out these changes and feelings in your own heads, but do it with your hands clasped together because, together, you are experiencing this major change.

"Honestly, stupid me, I didn't expect our lives to change much at all, we'd just be towing a kid around with us. I was shocked and angry at first about how much our lives and our relationship changed." -Leisel

Like the previous chapter's suggestion of having a discussion about new baby duties and responsibilities, have a conversation with your partner about the changes you feel now that your relationship includes a third person. Listen to what your spouse has to say too. If he is feeling jealous because you are spending so much time with the baby, or thinks you now feel more love for her, let him know that he is definitely important too. Even though we, as new mothers, might feel like this baby has rocked our world, your partner is experiencing some of that too. The life he had a few months ago, pre-baby, is now drastically different even if he might seem like he is not that affected. If anything, he might be feeling frustrated and impatient because a baby can take up so much of his wife's time. It is okay to feel that way. It is natural. Just acknowledge your partner and his feelings, and hopefully he can acknowledge yours too.

"At first it [having a baby] made things harder in my marriage. My focus shifted completely to baby care and being a mom, and I forgot to be much of a wife for a while. It took a while to figure out I had to multitask in that arena too." -Leisel

Having to remember to make time for baby, partner, and yourself is a very delicate balancing act. Someone will end up neglected (and it will probably be yourself), but just do your best. When your baby is very young and you are just starting to get the hang of caring for an infant most of your time will be consumed by baby care, but things will ease up. You will get to understand the flow of naps and down-time for your baby. You will know when you can lie her down and let her look at her mobile for awhile, then you can shift your focus to your husband or yourself. Try not to feel the weight of housework, relatives wanting to see the baby, or getting the baby pictures—it can all wait.

"Spending time alone without the baby and nurturing your marriage is crucial, even though it can be hard to do." -Teresa

13

Sleep Deprivation and Trade-offs

Let us acknowledge it here and now: Sleep deprivation is a form of torture. It truly is. Many of us have experienced nights with a few hours sleep due to school or work or just having too much fun, and it was a bit painful, but we made it up and recovered. That is nothing compared to night after night of little sleep and constant exhaustion (probably only med school could compare). You just do not feel like yourself when your body and your brain is lacking the necessary recovery time it needs from sleep; and not just one hour of sleep, I mean the uninterrupted time of continuous sleep when your brain actually goes through all sleep stages multiple times and you feel truly rested. The feelings caused by sleep deprivation can be excruciating and like nothing you experienced before.

Lack of sleep was one of the most surprising and agonizing aspects of a new baby for me, and I was completely ignorant about it before we had our daughter. I had a difficult time sleeping even before she came along, during pregnancy, either from feeling uncomfortable, not being able to sleep on my stomach, or just awake with heartburn or hunger. I developed an unwanted ritual of watching reruns of TV shows from the '80s and having peanut butter toast with a glass of milk at three in the morning in those last few months (and I wondered how I gained so much weight). My husband's grandmother always said that not being able to sleep while pregnant was preparation for a newborn: you are learning to deal with having interrupted or little sleep on a continual basis. I disagree. When you are pregnant and cannot sleep, you can nap during the weekends, you can lazily stare at the television if you want, you can take it easy all day and people have sympathy for you. Once you are a new mom with an infant, you do not get the luxury of having that down-time because you still have that baby to care for, even when you are completely drained and barely hanging in there. It is shocking at first when you realize that this little baby will need you again very soon (to eat, be changed, or soothed), whether you are ready for it or not.

"I was accepting of the responsibilities [of a new baby], I just think that it's an exhaustion that you can't fully explain to people. They have to go through it themselves to fully understand. I remember being worried while pregnant when I read that babies needed to eat every two or three hours and I thought, 'I'll never be able to do it. I need my sleep or I'll be a wreck.' Sometimes I was a bit of a wreck, but after she was born, I found that it was no longer all about me, but rather all about her. I found that helped make the sleeplessness and constant work more tolerable. But there were times when I just couldn't

give anymore, I HAD to sleep. Thankfully my husband helped a lot." -Teresa

When our daughter was a couple weeks old and we had just left her doctor's office after a check-up appointment, I remember looking through the free baby-care book they gave us and reading aloud to my husband the three short paragraphs about a baby's sleeping habits in the first six months. I was dismayed to learn that most babies will wake up every two to three hours to eat and that can last from birth to four months (or longer). Our daughter was a typical baby, starting with needing to eat every two hours then slowly stretching it out to three to four hours. We triumphed over every hour that she could go beyond. My husband and I would break the nights down into two shifts. Usually I went to bed early and took the first one that would go through one round of feeding, changing, and putting her back to bed, then at the second wake-up my husband would take over. I was glad that he could help in that way. I do not think I could have made it and stayed sane if he was not available to let me have a few hours of uninterrupted sleep.

Many breastfeeding moms take on the entire night duty and that is a job in itself, however there is always the option of pumping and letting your partner do some of the night feedings. You also can divide it up by feeding the baby then handing her off so that your partner does the changing and putting back to sleep. Just because the food comes from you does not mean that your husband has to be excluded from the night shift! Discuss it with him and find a system that works for both of you. Explain that you need sleep in order to function, feel somewhat normal, and be the best mom and wife you can be.

"I knew being a mom was a lot of work, but I did not realize how much. For example, the lack of sleep (only getting two hours) and the wear of always having to nurse." -Quinn

Our daughter did eventually stretch out to longer sleeping periods and my husband and I would trade off nights once she made it to only waking up once. I remember feeling overjoyed when she reached four months old and the doctor said she could start to eat rice cereal. I thought she would immediately start sleeping longer once she had solid (or less liquid) food in her belly. I was mistaken about that as well. The rice cereal did help, but it was not the magic key to sleeping longer. Growing, thriving, eating, and being a healthy baby was what made her sleep longer, and that takes time (along with learning when she is truly hungry at night or just waking up and a little fussy but able to go back to sleep).

My uncle jokingly warned me that at some point the baby will sleep continuously for seven or eight hours and when she does, I will wake up in a panic and wonder if she is okay. I joked and laughed with him when he said that, but, sure enough, he was right. One night she went from sleeping four or five hours to a complete eight and my husband and I both woke up, looked at the clock, realized that neither of us had gotten up with her that night, then rushed into the room to find her still sleeping! We were amazed. Of course, the next few nights she would back to waking up two or three times again and we wondered what had happened during that magical night of continuous sleep. She eventually did it again, and ever so slowly she worked up to sleeping through the night, most nights, by the time she was nine months old.

Those months of constant wakings, however, can really wear you down. A few times my mother-in-law graciously did the night feedings and let my husband and I sleep all night; however, it often seemed like getting a good night's sleep after continually not getting one only made us feel more tired, as though our bodies realized what was missing. There is no question that these first months can be agonizing, but here are a few ways to make it a little less painful.

Tips to Help Sleep Deprivation

1. Try to make up sleep if you can. This means taking naps when the baby does. I understand that it is not always possible. For instance, I could not sleep due to the pressure of trying to make myself sleep in a short amount of time! If that is the case, see number two below.

2. If you cannot nap, REST. This means just lying down and closing your eyes, playing relaxing music or a relaxation visualization, or anything that you find restful and giving your body and brain a chance to recover. Agree

with yourself that you will lie there for twenty minutes with your eyes closed, sleep or no sleep, to give your body a rest—no looking at your phone or any other screen (mute them all). Close your tired eyes and lay there. If you feel anxious doing this, do it anyway; it will pass.

3. Realize that it is temporary. Your baby eventually will make it to sleeping all night. Every baby is different, but yours will get there. When you feel like you can't take it any more, take a deep breath and know that this is a *temporary* time in your life. If you think your baby is waking up more than she should, consult a few books on baby sleep (there are many out there). One book that I found very helpful was *Good Night, Sleep Tight: The Sleep Lady's Gentle Guide to Helping Your Child Go to Sleep, Stay Asleep, and Wake Up Happy* by Kim West.

4. Do away with any "shoulds" (see Chapter 6 for help). For example, "I should do the dishes; I should do a load of laundry; I should call my friend back; I should check in at work." Just let all of this go for the time being. You will get back to doing all of these things, and more, but during this time while your baby is still very young and needy, give yourself a break from all of the chores and duties you usually do. For these first few months, just be.

5. Use Christina's advice on how to deal with little sleep:

"1. It'll be okay. You will get much more sleep in the relatively near future. Hang in there. 2. Smile. It makes you feel better. 3. Cry. It makes you feel better." -Christina

As your baby grows and you get to interact with him, he becomes more enjoyable—to see that cute toothless smile, to hear those coos, and to watch as he learns that he has toes (and, boy, do they taste good). And as you and your partner adjust to a new family member, life settles into a more comfortable existence. Not to say that it becomes easy, but it does change. There are trade-offs when you compare a newborn to a crawling explorer. When he is an infant he needs to eat often, and you might feel like you are constantly changing a diaper or trying to figure out why he is so fussy, but the benefit to this little being is that he stays in one place, and he can be entertained by a mobile or a toy hanging from a car seat. He is new to the world and often just looking outside is an incredible experience for him. You can safely do other things while he stares, fascinated by a fly on the screen door.

Then he grows and grows, and before you know it, he is crawling around on the kitchen floor and he has two teeth. He is fat and adorable. He sleeps longer and as a result, you do too. Life is improving on that front. You are starting to feel like "yourself" again. *But*...you cannot leave him alone for a minute. He is always on the go, he wants to see and feel (and taste) everything. It is so much fun to watch him learn and explore, but it can be exhausting too. What happened to those days of him lying on the floor and you going to the bathroom by yourself? These are the trade-offs of your growing baby. Life improves in one area, but becomes challenging in another. And so it goes. At the moment my children are nine and seven, and the life of trade-offs does not stop. They outgrow one phase only to move into another. But that is okay; they are growing and changing every day, and that is part of the process. One period of their lives might be easier than another—it all depends on the child and the parent. Some people enjoy toddlers and their zest for life; others find babies more to their liking; and yet others think it is better when they can walk and talk and ask for what they want. Sometimes they just surprise you by what they can do or say, and you find yourself laughing at their new-found ability to blow bubbles in their milk. Just know that if you are having a difficult time right now, it will slowly transition to a different phase. As my mother-in-law likes to point out when the kids are especially challenging, "Life isn't boring." And that is so true.

14

Day-to-Day Life While Working or Staying Home: The Need for Routine

As you settle in with a new baby, one of the most helpful and comforting ways to get used to this new part of life is to have a routine. Most of us are creatures of habit: we like things "just so" and feel uncomfortable when something new is added or taken away. As we know, a baby changes everything—from the way the house runs to the new outlook you have on seatbelt laws and terrorist sightings in Europe. Life is quite upside for a while as you and your partner, and other family members, adjust. Life does settle though, and you will find yourself slowing adapting to a new routine. You will come to know what time your baby typically wakes up in the morning, how often he gets hungry, if he has a particularly fussy time during the day, and slowly a pattern will develop.

You have the ability to shape this routine in certain ways. For instance, you go for a walk at 3:00 in the afternoon because your baby feels better in the stroller and this is his last nap of the day, or you feed him at 10:30 in the morning because he naps around 11:00. Your baby will dictate the schedule for the most part, but you both will get to know when certain things happen. A routine is helpful for everyone: you, your baby, and any other caregiver who might take over for a time. It is reliable and certain (most of the time) and lets your baby feel safe and reassured that he will be cared for in a dependable way. Some parents cringe at the idea of a routine, thinking it is too rigid and confining, but a routine is what you make of it. Everything does not need to happen exactly at the time you plan (and with a baby that is often not possible anyway); some days might be a little different, but a loose routine will help you get back to a semi-normal life after such a major change. If you have not set a schedule yet, watch your baby for cues. Although she is constantly changing, there are predictable times when she needs to eat, sleep, play, etc. From that you can shape one that works for both of you.

The hard part comes when, after you have adjusted to a new life and have this new routine set in place, you have to go back to work. Some mothers already made the decision to stay home with their babies and can continue with their routines as planned, but for many other new mothers, maternity leave is limited and they reach the inevitable time of returning to their jobs. This can be an incredibly difficult time for your family as everyone adjusts to yet another change, but a change is all it is and you will adapt to that one as well.

"It was hard at first. You always hear about how difficult it is to leave them for the first time, and my experience was no exception. I was comfortable with the daycare I found, but I still cried when I walked out the door without her the first time. Eventually, I was glad to be back to work. I feel the time she spends in daycare benefits her, and I benefit being productive at my job and socializing as well. I feel I have the best of both worlds, but I am able to only work two days a week." -Teresa

All mothers handle this back-to-work transition differently. For some it is heart-wrenching, they have their new little babies and are loath to part with them. This is understandable. Even if you do not think you have fully bonded to your baby, once you have to leave him every day to go to work, you suddenly have a much different view than you had before giving birth. Now, you want to be with him every minute of every day. These are normal feelings, and do not make yourself feel worse by telling yourself to get over it. It hurts, acknowledge it, but know it is a grieving process that you will get through in time. Most of the women in the mothers' group had to return to work; they had no choice financially, and that is often the case. So cry all that you need to, hug your baby for an hour when you get home, and allow those painful feelings to come because they will eventually pass.

One new mom I recently met went back to work and had a very tough time doing it. She is a teacher and confessed that she would cry in the bathroom at lunch and on breaks. It was just so hard to leave her daughter, even though she was comfortable with the caregiver she hired. She said that the first week was the worst, but that it slowly got easier. She has said that it helps to think that she and her husband are both working for their daughter, in order to provide her with things that they otherwise could not afford if only one person worked. That is a good way to look at an otherwise painful situation.

"It was kind of hard. I started a new job after staying home for the first six months. My husband stays home with her, which made it easier. Pumping was hard and I was tired a lot. But pumping also gave me a chance to take a few good breaks during the workday, which was helpful. I felt guilty being away from her so much, but needed to learn to trust my husband more. He does a really good job and when I get home from work, I have renewed 'kid' energy to really spend quality time with her (most of the time)." -Christina

After you start to adjust to this new transition, you will begin to see some of the benefits like Christina does. More than likely, after you get home for the day, you will want to spend as much time with that baby as you can. Your son will get your undivided attention, which he loves, and you will truly want to spend time with him, not just feel like you should. He will be excited to see you and you will feel the same (hopefully, unless it was a really long and stressful day). Work also gives back dimensions of your life that you put on hold for a while—for many it provides a mental aspect and social one as well. Ideally, you like your job and the people you work with, so returning might make life more "complete."

"My job is unique in that I'm a pediatric nurse at a university hospital. I love exercising my mind, having the social outlet, and experiencing a rewarding career." -Kelley

One mom I knew, who had a very demanding newborn (colic and extreme fussiness), was relieved to return to work. She said that she loves her daughter, of course, and was glad that she and her husband had her, but it created such turmoil in their lives for a while, especially within their marriage, that going back to work and finding that routine again really suited all of them. Remember that it is okay to enjoy your job and still be a great mom! Finding a balance and thriving because of it will benefit your baby and your family.

On the flipside of that are the stay-at-home moms who made the choice to be full-time mothers. This is a difficult transition as well. Many women worked full time before they had their babies and now they are facing the life of staying at home, all day, every day. Feelings of isolation and loneliness can arise from this daily existence if you are not careful to take into account all of your needs—a social outlet, mental stimulation, etc. Many of us face feelings of unworthiness for being "just a mom." And yet many of us also know how ridiculous this is: moms have one of the hardest and most important jobs in the world. But for some reason, many of us feel like we are looked down upon for dedicating our lives, full time, to motherhood.

"I knew that I wanted to stay at home with my baby from the start and that has never changed. However, I often wish I had a job to escape to. I feel less worthy just being a stay-at-home mother and often feel that I am looked down upon by family and friends." -Tanya

I have felt the same way Tanya does. I went back to work for two days a week after I had my children. I was fortunate to have family watch my babies while I went to work. And even though I had a job, I considered myself more a "mom" than anything else. I was more focused on caring for these two little beings than advancing a career, and that is okay (though it still can be hard to accept).

Recently, however, when I was at a family birthday party, a high-powered working woman I had never met began the conversation with the inevitable question, "What do you do?" I paused, wondering how to answer her question, knowing that I could not honestly say that I was a federal judge or some equally important sounding profession, so I said, "Uh, well, I'm a mom mostly," pointing to my two young children. She seemed to soften just slightly after that and moved on to interrogating my husband about his career choice. This woman obviously defined herself and others based on what they did for a living and not for who they are as people, which is her own shortcoming, and yet I could not help but feel cross-examined and somewhat "less than" because my answer was "I am a mom," period, with no other titles or answers beyond that. Obviously, I am more than "just a mom" and so are the millions of other women who have children; we were all "something" before we had babies (women, human beings), but for some reason we feel the need to define ourselves by our jobs. The next time someone asks me, "What do you do?" I think I might just answer, "Lots of things." Whether you have gone back to work or stay at home with your baby, do not let either decision define you, you are much more than that.

"As a career woman, I always thought I would go back to work within a few months. In fact, it took me about seven to eight months to admit I was a stay-at-home mom. This has been a very difficult career change, since my job had been so much a part of how I defined myself and who I was." -Kristen

15

Views on Moms:
We Are That Strong

"I don't think I really had a view of mothers before I had my own child. Of course, we all had our own mothers and knew many others, but I never really paid attention to that role. I was a career woman and was striving to make it in the business world—I didn't really think about being a mother as a career choice." -Kristen

The decision to become a mother is obviously a serious one, whether your pregnancy came intentionally or by surprise. You are taking on the responsibility of being someone's mom, which is massive in weight. And yet, motherhood is such a common role in our society that most people do not think much of it, most of the time. Now that we have all entered the realm of being moms, it helps to think about how we once thought of these people with their kids at their heels, because, let's face it, we are now one of them.

"I thought mothers, or at least the mom I would become, were the ultimate picture of balance. I didn't base this idea on any one person, but on a collective view of the suburban mom, going to the gym, carting kids to school and practices, making brownie treats, and keeping the house together and being ready for the next meal or potluck..." -Teresa

Teresa's imagined scene of motherhood sounds ideal, and it would be nice if it were that easy, but as we all now know, it is not. Being a mother is hard work (as this entire book shows), and too often society does not place enormous value on the role of being a good mother—one who cares, who tries, who fails, who learns, who tries again, and who loves completely. We must make the effort to honor ourselves and other mothers in the world. We are attempting to raise children who care about the world and everyone in it (hopefully), but we must have our own lives in this balance too. We cannot completely dedicate our lives to anyone or thing because we will then lose ourselves in the process. We must be true to ourselves while acknowledging that we play a very important role in the world. Whether you see it as mundane or not, as moms, we make a very big difference to those in our lives.

"We are a diverse group. I just wish all moms had the resources to really care for their children with less stress. Moms, like everyone else, should think before they act, which we could all work on a little. I also think the role isn't taken as seriously as it should be—mothers have such a huge impact on the people

their children will become in the world. I know that who I am was largely formed by my mother's daily work in my life."
-Christina

And because we have taken on this role of being a mother, we are strong. Growing a baby and giving birth is beautiful and truly is a miracle, but it is an incredibly hard experience, on your body, brain, and spirit. You gave a piece of yourself to create this being, and that is no small thing. For some of us, the labor and delivery of these amazing babies was almost more than we could bear. I did not think that I had such strength in me during the birth of my first child.

A friend who recently had an even longer labor than mine, which ended with exhaustion, tears, and an emergency C-section, was shocked and angry after the birth of her baby. She thought that the doctor could have prevented many of the issues she faced during labor. I explained to her that no one can change what the doctor decided, and hopefully he chose the best path (in his medical opinion). Then I said, "but think about how strong you are. Did you ever think you could have taken on something like this? No one ever wants an overly painful and traumatic labor and birth, but you have probably learned more about yourself during this experience than you ever thought you could know. Something that you probably would never have known if you had not gone through it." She thought about that and agreed. "I never thought I could have done anything close to that before I had this baby," she said. "People may never know how hard it was for me, but at least I know that I did it." "Exactly," I told her. "You are stronger than you know."

"I think moms could lighten up on themselves a little. It's hard work raising a family today, and the pressure we put on ourselves doesn't make it any easier." -Teresa

Another mother that I met in the moms' group had twins. We were all in awe of her for even showing up at a mom's group with *two* babies in tow. She would come in pushing her double stroller and carefully lay out two blankets and take out each baby girl and lay her down. The mom looked neat and calm (whereas I believed that if I had two babies, I would show up in rumpled clothes with my hair standing up and my make-up half done). We all admired her and thought that she must be so much better at this than we were. And yet, after getting to know her, she revealed that she had a very difficult time adjusting to having babies. There were times when they were all crying together, she told me, and she did not know if she could make it through the day. She told me that her mother was supposed to help her after the births, but that her grandmother was having some medical problems at the time so her mother went to help her grandmother instead. She was very angry about that. She thought that her mother should have come to assist her with these two new little babies, and that her grandmother was seeking attention because her medical issues were not that serious.

I sympathized with her because, again, in that moment I could not imagine caring for *two* newborns. But I also told her that her mother's absence forced her to be stronger because she had no other choice. She had to dig a little deeper and go through a very difficult time, but in the end, she learned that she *could* do it. She was that strong. And we all are. We try each day to do the best for our families, and that is not easy. Our jobs as moms are continuous; and even when we are at work or having a night out, our thoughts do not stop concerning the well-being of our children. We are one hundred percent committed to this job, and we should commend ourselves for taking on this challenging role and showing up every day.

"Being a mother is a wonderful blessing. But, society and our own conflicting views often gets in our way of being the best mom we can be. Motherhood is the hardest thing I have ever done, but also the most rewarding." -Tanya

Another friend of mine has four daughters. They are all grown now and she has the pleasure of being a grandmother. But during the midst of her young motherhood, the last baby came as a complete surprise (her husband had a vasectomy and she still got pregnant). Her story took me aback. I could not imagine having another baby, especially after having three, and thinking that pregnancies and infants were a thing of the past. I told her that I didn't think I would have made it if that happened to me. She said that I would have, because you "just do." I understood what she meant: in difficult times when you do not think you can go any more or handle another minute, you "just do" because you have to, because you have a baby who needs to be comforted, because your three-year-old has the stomach flu in the middle of the night and is scared, because your child ends up in the emergency room, whatever the case is: when it comes to being a mother, you "just do" and know that you will get through this time. Yes, we all need to recover, we all need down-time, and time to process and reflect, but in the midst of all of it, you "just do," and know that it will all be okay.

So as you get to know this baby in your arms and start to see his personality emerge, as he wows you with rolling over, and melts your heart with his smiles, know that *you* are his mother. You are important and strong and one of the greatest forces in your baby's life. You matter more than you know. And though you are facing some difficult times and part of you never thought that you would be here in this moment, while another part of you might think you won't get through the hard times, know that you will. You are that strong. You and your new family are growing together and learning from each other each day. Follow in the footsteps of millions of mothers over thousands of years and know that you are part of something important and life changing. When it gets harder and you are exhausted and closer to the edge than you ever thought possible, just close your eyes and take a breath. You can do this. We all know you can.

PART THREE: *Coping Strategies*

Questions to Consider from Part Three:

One of the most helpful things I learned to do for myself is to reflect upon my big experiences and write about them. Journaling helps me to clear away the buildup of emotions, feelings, fears, judgments, and whatever else is swirling around in my subconscious. I recommend reading through these questions and writing about them, but the choice is yours. Sometimes, just reading and thinking about them will be enough to help you make some realizations that you were not consciously aware of before. And those insights will help you process your experience, transition more easily into your new life, and help you to remember it better—because the first year of having your baby will drift away in a fog before you know it.

1) What were some things that you liked to do during your free time before your baby came along? Make a list. Have you been able to do any of these things since having your baby? Do you miss them?

2) Are there any local support groups in your area? If you don't know, search local hospitals or churches to see. Would you consider attending a new mothers' support group? Why or why not?

3) Do you have family or friends who help out with your baby? Do you feel comfortable asking others for help?

Make a list of people you can go to if needed.

4) Is your spouse or partner supportive? What does he do to help you with the baby? Do you think he should do more, or less? Think up a way to have a conversation about it without accusing or placing blame. Write out some possible starting points.

5) What are some common interests that you and your partner share? What did you like to do together, pre-baby? Name at least three things.

6) Have you had a discussion with your partner about how he is feeling with the change of a baby in your lives? Does he think things have changed? Ask him.

7) Do you think that you are suffering from exhaustion or being overtired all of the time? What are some ways to help yourself get more sleep or rest during this difficult period? Make a list.

8) If you are going back to work, or have already, are there any aspects of it that you are looking forward to? Are there any parts of your working life that you have missed? Try to focus on these instead of the pain of leaving your baby.

9) If you are staying home now full time, are you comfortable with that decision? Would you want to work?

(Any answer is acceptable; this is your life.) Do you ever feel judged for being a stay-at-home mom?

10) Taking away the struggles, exhaustion, and possible physical or mental pain, how has your experience of motherhood been for you? Do you see yourself as an important person in the eyes of your baby? Know that you are. Write a letter to your son or daughter telling him or her how this experience has been, and how it has changed your life. Keep it and look at it every few years to remind yourself of how it was when you had your baby. Save it and share it with him or her twenty years from now, your grown-up "baby."

16

Advice for New Moms

Following is advice for new moms from those who participated in this book:

"Always be thankful for what you have. I know that can be relative, considering struggles and health issues we all may encounter, but there's always something to appreciate. Rely on others. Don't be afraid to ask for help, because it's surprising how much friends and family will want to help but just don't want to interfere. You don't need to read a zillion books—just go with what seems to make common sense. Do what feels right to you, not based on others' comments or rules." -Kelley

"Learn to take a deep breath, a break and/or a nap whenever you can. Those spider webs aren't going anywhere, play with your kid, they grow up too fast and when you blink you miss something. If the diaper really explodes and you just can't deal with it, don't be afraid to cut off the outfit and throw it away. Sometimes it just isn't worth washing that out!" -Leisel

"Accept help from anyone who is willing to give it. Learn

to count to ten slowly… this too shall pass. There is no right or wrong way. Do what works for you and your baby." -Tanya

"While you are pregnant, spend more time with your friends who are already moms so you can get a better view into the new life that will be yours soon." -Kristen

"It seemed like people knew a lot of details about what their kids needed, which I struggled with as we went from phase to phase of development. There is a LOT of discovery the first year. I learned that you do just kind of figure it out as you go along, and a lot of effective parenting is a combination of my own personality, my husband's personality, and my daughter's personality (i.e., what works for us won't work for everyone else, and vice versa). However, I will temper that last sentence by saying how much I appreciated ideas on the myriad of baby-care issues I needed, and continue to need, help with. It gave me a lot of things to try, some of which worked! I knew it would be fun to be a mom, but I also heard it was a lot of work…" -Christina

"I would have spent more time connecting with moms in the beginning. I was too fearful my baby was crying too much and people didn't want us around. At the same time I would have stayed home more. I would have written down more milestones." -Kelley

"I am glad that I got to be a part of the mommy club. I do have to say now that I am a mom that it is truly a full-time job.

Motherhood is the best gift I could have asked for and I would not change a thing. Motherhood is a true hands-on learning experience. You get a little dirty, literally, to learn." -Quinn

"1. Follow your instincts. 2. Remember to laugh. Trust me, it'll be funny later. 3. Try not to compare...your weight gain, your baby's milestones... A new mother is beautiful and your baby is a blessing." -Renée

"There's no such thing as perfection—just do the best you can and that's good enough. Keep your sense of humor! Savor this time and enjoy every moment." -Lory

"Really enjoy your old life of picking up at the drop of a hat to go to dinner, shopping, or vacation. Expect the unexpected; know that every baby is different and don't be afraid to try anything. You need to do what works for your baby and try not to listen to negative advice on what you should be doing. In the beginning you are in survival mode, and that is okay. The first eight to twelve weeks will be tough; be aware that it does get better." -Nancy

"1. Love God with all your heart and he will help you through any situation. 2. Realize that you don't know all the answers and seek advice from other experienced mommies. 3. When things get tough, just remind yourself that you will make it through and enjoy the time you spend with your kids." -Amy

"1. Take naps with the little one. 2. Take lots of pictures; even if you don't put them in a scrapbook they are great to look back on. 3. Take time out for yourself. Being a mommy you sometimes forget about yourself. Try to take time out to do something nice. A quiet bath, time to read, paint your toes, or a savory yummy treat." -Quinn

"Capture it and write it down. Take a picture, make a note about that day, make a list of funny things that have happened with your baby or things you have learned about yourself. Before you know it, three years then five years then ten years will have passed and you will look back and fail to remember all of those little moments. Do your future self a favor, and start today." -Jennifer

A Letter to New Dads

Dear new Dad,

Does that word have a strange sound to you? Dad, father, papa, pops there are many names to go by, but in the beginning this new title might sound and feel a little weird. You're a new dad, you have a new baby, and your wife or partner is now a mother. What monumental changes can happen in what feels like such a short time! (Or a long time depending on how pregnancy and birth went.) Either way, you have a new family member and a new family. Congratulations! These are times you will never forget.

Maybe you're still in shock about this new being who has come into your world. Maybe you feel love in a way you never felt before. Or maybe you're exhausted and confused about how things will change and how your wife has changed too. All of these feelings (anything you're feeling) is okay. Even if you think that nothing is different and it's back to work on Monday, that's okay too.

But know, for better or worse (we'll say for better), much has changed and will continue to, especially over the next few months, and the year. A baby (or babies) can and will transform almost everything in our lives. We learn to adapt to their needs—their feedings, their naps, their fast developing bodies and brains. It is truly amazing when you stop and think about it, but it also can be overwhelming and frustrating, and even depressing sometimes.

Know that this new upturned world will eventually even out. Your new family will develop a rhythm and a routine. It won't be chaotic forever. Also know that your wife has a new full-time job that is non-stop, twenty four hours a day, seven days a week and she would appreciate your support, although she may not say it or ask for it. Going through pregnancy and birth is stressful on a woman's body and spirit. So please be patient as she adjusts, her hormones equilibrate, and she learns about the new and weighty responsibilities of being a new mom. It will take some time; know that she still loves you, probably even more now that you two share this amazing baby who is part of you both (even if he or she is adopted, you are both equally influential).

Giving your wife a break in the form of an afternoon out or just a nap by herself will also give you the opportunity of getting to know your new son or daughter. Dads are just as important in a new baby's life. Don't be afraid to get in there and help; your wife will appreciate it (even if she can't show it right now). As you both adjust to this new life with a baby, hopefully you both will make the effort to be patient, kind, and supportive of each other. That is difficult to do when exhaustion sets in and the daily grind of a baby's needs must be met, but take a deep breath and know this time truly is temporary. The adjustment to living with a baby can be hard for moms and dads, but you are both in it together. And if you feel a little neglected or left out, know that your wife will be back and be the person you remember and love. It might take a little time, but it will happen.

So try to take this time to be present, to find the humor, to find the good, and keep reminding yourself that it will all be okay and life will continue to change. Your baby will grow (probably before you know it), and he or she will be crawling then walking and talking, and giggling and having all sorts of fun, probably making you laugh while infuriating you all at the same time. You get to witness and be a part of it all. The days are long, but the years are short. Welcome to fatherhood! It is sure to be a wild and memorable ride.

Warmly,
Once a New Mom

~ 17 ~

Full Questionnaires with Answers

Below is the questionnaire used to guide the writing of this book, along with the complete answers from all of the moms who participated. They might be helpful to you.

Quinn

1) What was your view of mothers and motherhood before you had your own child?

I envied all the moms. I really wanted to be one. I thought what a cool job it would be. To have a child to love, take care of, and see grow through the years.

2) Did you always think you would be a mom, or was the idea of children a changing one?

I always thought I would be a mom. When we were trying to conceive and it did not happen I was very depressed. I finally had to go on fertility drugs and IT WORKED!! Yeah, I was so excited and shocked when the doctor finally said the wonderful words, "You are pregnant."

3) What were your first thoughts and feelings after you had your baby?

My first thoughts... nothing, really. I remember having tears come out of my eyes when they held her up for the first time and it feeling so surreal. I remember not wanting to let her out of my arms. It was very calming holding her. I also remember thinking that is was a weird feeling having a baby nurse on me. They asked if I was going to nurse. I said yes and all of a sudden I was naked and nursing. I looked down and my heart melted.

4) Was it hard to believe initially that you were actually a mom? Please explain.

It was hard to believe. I was so excited during my pregnancy to see my little one. But after I gave birth and they placed her on my chest it was surreal. I couldn't wrap my brain around that I was a mom. It was weird but exciting and a joy all in one.

5) When did you really start feeling like you were a mother? Was it during pregnancy, right after the birth, or did it happen later?

I felt like a mother when I looked down (after giving birth) to a cute naked nursing baby on my chest.

6) Did you immediately bond with your baby or did it take a little time? If it did take some time, about how long?

I think I bonded immediately with Molly. It was an amazing experience giving birth and then seeing her brought tears to my eyes. It still does :-)

7) Did you find it hard to accept the new responsibilities that a baby brought? Please explain.

Truthfully?? Yes. I knew being a mom was a lot of work but I did not realize how much. For example, the lack of sleep (only getting two hours) and the wear of always having to nurse.

8) Did you have support (other than a spouse or partner) or seek it out?

My husband, Paul, was great. He was very supportive through the pregnancy and birth. He is the one I have to thank for keeping me in shape while pregnant, and for being there and helping me through the birth. Even though I scared him when it was time. He thought I was a burglar.

9) Did having a child change your marriage or your relationship with your partner either positively or negatively? Please explain and/or give examples.

It changed both ways. Positive, because it brought us closer together. Negatively, because now that she is older it is hard to have "us" time. With busy work schedules and crazy hours. It is a treat when she falls asleep early.

10) If it did change, were you surprised about this?

Not really. I figured with having a kid that things would change and not be the same as when it was just the two of us.

11) Do you work or stay at home?
Work full-time.

12) If you work, how did you cope with the change of going back to work? Was it hard to do? What is it a relief to get back to a routine? What helped you?

Besides crying?? It was the hardest thing I had to do. I did not want to leave my baby. I felt like a horrible mom that I was abandoning her. I cried all the time. I went at lunch to nurse her and still go and hang out on my lunch break. But when I went back to work I felt like I was missing out on everything. I did not want to miss a moment or a milestone. I missed a few and I was upset about that. Thank goodness I did not miss the first steps. The things that helped me besides visiting at lunch was taking pictures and putting them up on my computer and frames around the office. Also, I tried to take it one day at a time and transition back in to work slowly. That did not last due to finances. But it was nice working four instead of five days. One day made a huge difference.

14) What would you have done differently if you could do it all over again (this answer can cover anything from coming home from the hospital to taking a weekend away to making decisions about your baby)?

I would have taken more time off work before Molly was born. Also, leave earlier from the recovery part of the hospital. We tried but they lagged. I hated that part. It was hard they just left you there. No one came in to bring water or anything. Thank goodness for family.

15) Do you find yourself ever feeling like the guilty mommy (for any reason)? If so, how do you cope with this?

I felt so guilty and horrible for leaving to go to work. I cried myself to work for two months and on my nursing breaks. I still feel a little guilty, but I know that I am doing a good thing. Maybe one day I can stay home with her or work part time. That's the goal. I also felt guilty for missing out on milestones because I was at work.

16) Do you think society portrays a certain image of mothers that we all must aspire to? If so, what is that image and do you think it's possible (or necessary) to become that mom?

I don't think so.

17) What would be three pieces of advice (practical, inspirational, etc.) that you would give first-time moms?

1. Take naps with the little one. 2. Take lots of pictures even if you don't put them in a scrapbook, they are great to look back on. 3. Take time out for yourself. Being a mommy you sometimes forget about yourself. Try to take time out to do something nice. A quiet bath, time to read, paint your toes, or a savory yummy treat.

18) What is your view of mothers and motherhood today?

The same, I am glad that I get to be a part of the mommy club. I do have to say, now that I am a mom, that it is truly a full-time job. Motherhood is the best gift I could have asked for and [I] would not change a thing.

Motherhood is a true hands-on learning experience. You get a little dirty, literally, to learn.

Any other comments you wish to make?
Motherhood is the best gift I could have asked for and [I] would not change a thing.

Christina

1) What was your view of mothers and motherhood before you had your own child?

It seemed like people knew a lot of details about what their kids needed, which I struggled with as we went from phase to phase of development. There is a LOT of discovery the first year. I learned that you do just kind of figure it out as you go along, and a lot of effective parenting is a combination of my own personality, my husband's personality and my daughter's personality (i.e., what works for us won't work for everyone else and vice versa). However, I will temper that last sentence by saying how much I appreciated ideas on the myriad of baby-care issues I needed and continue to need help with. It gave me a lot of things to try, some of which worked! I knew it would be fun to be a mom, but I also heard it was a lot of work...

2) Did you always think you would be a mom, or was the idea of children a changing one?

I always thought I would be a mother in some way, shape, or form—either through birth, adoption, as a teacher, or some combination of these.

3) What were your first thoughts and feelings after you had your baby?

I want to go to sleep. And "Can someone help me nurse?" And "My pelvis really hurts." And "I really want to sleep." And before the first cry, "Is she OK?" That was a scary moment—that moment of waiting to hear the first cry.

4) Was it hard to believe initially that you were actually a mom? Please explain.

It was. But I felt like I just kind of got busy taking care of her constant needs. Is she eating? Is she sleeping? Is she looking around? Does she need a diaper change? Did she poop? How much? What did it look like? There was little time for reflection on motherhood for me...

5) When did you really start feeling like you were a mother? Was it during pregnancy, right after the birth, or did it happen later?

I think I started feeling like a mother in the first few weeks when I became the expert on this little person. I knew her routine and what she needed when better than anyone else. I was the only one who could provide certain things for her and that made me feel like she was mine. I also felt pretty mother-y during pregnancy. I would chat with her while she was in the womb, telling her what we would do when she was born, how it hurt my ribs when she stretched that way. It was fun, feeling like she was getting to know my voice.

6) Did you immediately bond with your baby or did it take a little time? If it did take some time, about how long?

I remember being kind of teary and again, being swept up in meeting her initial needs. I just wanted her to be okay, so most of my thoughts were about nursing, poop, and sleeping toward the beginning. I can't remember feeling un-bonded with her, so I guess it happened (if "it" is a singular event) pretty soon after her birth.

7) Did you find it hard to accept the new responsibilities that a baby brought? Please explain.

YES! After seven years of marriage and career, it was a challenge for me to give up the simple things I liked to do for myself, like reading magazines. Free time just vanished and I don't know if anything could have really prepared me for the reality of that. I comforted myself by remembering that this was a season of life and at other times I would have lots of free time and probably wish I had kids around.

8) Did you have support (other than a spouse or partner) or seek it out?

I went to a new moms' group, which was invaluable in providing a support network. It was like a big brainstorming session on everything from gas to diaper rash to marital relationships. I would encourage any new mom to seek out a group. It was good to get out and talk with other people who actually wanted to hear me talk about baby stuff. I also had a lot of help from friends and people in my church.

9) Did having a child change your marriage or your relationship with your partner either positively or negatively? Please explain and/or give examples.

We already had a really solid relationship to begin with, which made things a lot easier when the stress and exhaustion of navigating a newborn came. We were both really supportive of each other and quick to forgive if one of us snapped. I was pretty laid up with a pelvic injury during birth for the first few months, and my husband stepped up with no complaints and really took care of both of us.

11) Do you work or stay at home?
Work full-time.

12) If you work, how did you cope with the change of going back to work? Was it hard to do? What is it a relief to get back to a routine? What helped you?

It was kind of hard. I started a new job after staying home for the first six months. My husband stays home with her, which made it easier. Pumping was hard and I was tired a lot. But pumping also gave me a chance to take a few good breaks during the workday, which was helpful. I felt guilty being away from her so much, but needed to learn to trust my husband more. He does a really good job and when I get home from work, I have renewed "kid" energy to really spend quality time with her (most of the time).

14) What would you have done differently if you could do it all over again (this answer can cover anything from coming home from the hospital to taking a weekend away to making decisions about your baby)?

I wouldn't have let her fall off the bed! I would've said no to more things because sometimes I just needed to stay home and rest and pushed myself too hard. I would also have not gone back to work until she was a year old, so the nursing/pumping thing could have possibly gone a little better. However, it might have been harder for her to transition to me being away at work at an older age...

15) Do you find yourself ever feeling like the guilty mommy (for any reason)? If so, how do you cope with this?

Sometimes I feel guilty for being competitive as a mother—like wanting my kid to reach milestones before others. What's that all about? It's very silly. All kids develop at their own rates, and the great majority turn out just fine! I also want to give her exposure to everything, which is impossible.

16) Do you think society portrays a certain image of mothers that we all must aspire to? If so, what is that image and do you think it's possible (or necessary) to become that mom?

I am jealous of moms who do nice crafty things, like

perfect party favors and fancy cakes. I'm just not a crafty person. There's quite a lot of pressure for moms to be smart, sexy, loving, and creative. It's a tall order.

17) What would be three pieces of advice (practical, inspirational, etc.) that you would give first-time moms?
 1. It'll be okay. You will get much more sleep in the relatively near future. Hang in there. 2. Smile. It makes you feel better. 3. Cry. It makes you feel better.

18) What is your view of mothers and motherhood today?
 We are a diverse group. I just wish all moms had the resources to really care for their children with less stress. Moms, like everyone else, should think before they act, which we could all work on a little. I also think the role isn't taken as seriously as it should be—mothers have such a huge impact on the people their children will become in the world. I know that who I am was largely formed by my mother's daily work in my life.

Any other comments you wish to make?
 I love the opportunity to reflect honestly about the experience of early motherhood. I hope this book is a valuable resource to many new moms.

Renée

1) What was your view of mothers and motherhood before you had your own child?
 I always knew that I wanted to be a mother. When

people asked me "What do you want to be when you grow up?" being a mother was my dream job.

2) Did you always think you would be a mom, or was the idea of children a changing one?

I always knew that I'd be a mother. It was something I expressed to my husband before we married that was an important part of who I was and am.

3) What were your first thoughts and feelings after you had your baby?

Overwhelming. Point blank. I never had baby blues or postpartum, but I had so many hands helping. My family, my in-laws...and all I wanted was to be alone with my daughter and refocus. Too many chiefs and not enough Indians, so to speak.

4) Was it hard to believe initially that you were actually a mom? Please explain.

I still don't believe it. And it won't be so until she says "Mommy." So technically, I STILL don't feel like a mom yet! (She's only eight months old.)

5) When did you really start feeling like you were a mother? Was it during pregnancy, right after the birth, or did it happen later?

See #4. I tease my husband that I feel like "The Keeper of the Baby," not her Mommy.

6) Did you immediately bond with your baby or did it take a little time? If it did take some time, about how long?

No, not immediately. It took a while. My daughter was very fussy and cried more than most babies (from what I've been told). It was hard to develop that bond when I was sleep-deprived, impatient, emotional, and completely overwhelmed. I'd say it took a few weeks.

7) Did you find it hard to accept the new responsibilities that a baby brought? Please explain.

Never. I knew that she was the most important thing in my life and I never second-guessed any sacrifice.

8) Did you have support (other than a spouse or partner) or seek it out?

I had more support than I needed. I learned quickly to nod politely and say "thank you." Then do whatever I felt was right. Following my own instincts was always the right path.

9) Did having a child change your marriage or your relationship with your partner either positively or negatively? Please explain and/or give examples.

I tease my husband..."The love has shifted!" He adores his little girl, and it is so special that it brings me to tears. He walks in the door at night and it's her that he runs to kiss first. And that is SO okay with me. I do the same thing.

10) If it did change, were you surprised about this?
No. We were ready to start a family.

11) Do you work or stay at home?
Stay at home.

13) If you stay at home, are you comfortable with this decision? Do you enjoy being a stay-at-home mom or do you sometimes wish that you had a job to go to. Do you sometimes feel that you should have a job (other than being a mom)?

I feel blessed to be able to stay home with my daughter. Most women would love to do so. It's tough on us financially, and I'm trying to find part-time work from home. But again, she is worth the sacrifice. If I had to go back to a full-time work week and put her in daycare, my heart would break. I can't imagine someone else seeing her first steps and hearing her first words.

14) What would you have done differently if you could do it all over again (this answer can cover anything from coming home from the hospital to taking a weekend away to making decisions about your baby)?

No regrets.

15) Do you find yourself ever feeling like the guilty mommy (for any reason)? If so, how do you cope with this?

It can sometimes be hard to keep your temper and lose control or become impatient. Especially when your baby is crying. When this happens to me, I sometimes feel guilty. It's not her fault. She doesn't have another way to communicate and humor has gotten me out of many situations. Laughter is truly the best medicine.

16) Do you think society portrays a certain image of mothers that we all must aspire to? If so, what is that image and do you think it's possible (or necessary) to become that mom?

Nobody is perfect. Not me. Not you. Not your mother. And not your mother-in-law, no matter what she says! You can only do what you think is best and make the decisions that work best for your family. Again, follow your instincts.

17) What would be three pieces of advice (practical, inspirational, etc.) that you would give first-time moms?

1. Follow your instincts. 2. Remember to laugh. Trust me, it'll be funny later. 3. Try not to compare...your weight gain, your baby's milestones...a new mother is beautiful and your baby is a blessing.

18) What is your view of mothers and motherhood today?

It can be whatever we choose it to be, as long as we respect each other's choices.

Lory M.

1) What was your view of mothers and motherhood before you had your own child?

How can this woman have so much control over other people's lives and tell them what they can and can't do?? She has so much power! (This was me thinking about my mother when I was a child.)

2) Did you always think you would be a mom, or was the idea of children a changing one?
Always hoped I'd be and I was.

3) What were your first thoughts and feelings after you had your baby?
Having my daughter was the happiest day of my life, to this day! That was my first thought. Second thought was, "Man, that really hurt!"

4) Was it hard to believe initially that you were actually a mom? Please explain.
For sure, this beautiful little creature came out of me?!?

5) When did you really start feeling like you were a mother? Was it during pregnancy, right after the birth, or did it happen later?
Immediately after giving birth, as I will for the rest of my life.

6) Did you immediately bond with your baby or did it take a little time? If it did take some time, about how long?
I felt a strong bond from the first time I held her!

7) Did you find it hard to accept the new responsibilities that a baby brought? Please explain.

My mother lived nearby which helped a great deal, since there was so much to learn. I've always loved being a mother.

8) Did you have support (other than a spouse or partner) or seek it out?

Mom, Dad, sister.

9) Did having a child change your marriage or your relationship with your partner either positively or negatively? Please explain and/or give examples.

No answer given.

10) If it did change, were you surprised about this?

No answer given.

11) Do you work or stay at home?

Work full-time.

12) If you work, how did you cope with the change of going back to work? Was it hard to do? What is it a relief to get back to a routine? What helped you?

I hated going back to work!! My daughter was born in August and by November I was back to work full time and she was in a daycare. I never got to see her first steps!

14) What would you have done differently if you could do

it all over again (this answer can cover anything from coming home from the hospital to taking a weekend away to making decisions about your baby)?

No answer given.

15) Do you find yourself ever feeling like the guilty mommy (for any reason)? If so, how do you cope with this?

No answer given.

16) Do you think society portrays a certain image of mothers that we all must aspire to? If so, what is that image and do you think it's possible (or necessary) to become that mom?

No answer given.

17) What would be three pieces of advice (practical, inspirational, etc) that you would give first time moms?

There's no such thing as perfection, just do the best you can and that's good enough. Keep your sense of humor! Savor this time and enjoy every moment.

18) What is your view of mothers and motherhood today?

There are no bratty children, just uneducated, undisciplined parents!

Nancy

1) What was your view of mothers and motherhood before you had your own child?

I don't think that I really gave them the full respect

that they deserved. I felt like my career was far more of a priority than any mom's job would be. I didn't know all that was involved with being a mom. Now I truly stand corrected, because it is one of the hardest jobs in the world.

2) Did you always think you would be a mom, or was the idea of children a changing one?

I always knew that I would be a mom, but I did not realize how much I would change as a person. The old me is a distant memory and sometimes I still wish I still had a little bit of the old me.

3) What were your first thoughts and feelings after you had your baby?

My first thought was "Thank you, Jesus, she is healthy and perfect." For nine months I stressed out about everything and now she is here. My next thought was "Man, I am tired and I do not have it in me tonight to take care of her." Then reality set in and I thought, "Oh boy, were we ready for this?"

4) Was it hard to believe initially that you were actually a mom? Please explain.

Yes, again for nine months I tried to prepare myself, but can you really ever prepare yourself? I kinda felt like I was still a kid and I still needed to be taken care of and now I was responsible for someone else's life. I mean, was the hospital really going to let my husband and I leave with this baby...are we supposed to take a test or have a background check...are you sure we can take her??? I am not so sure if we are qualified.

5) When did you really start feeling like you were a mother? Was it during pregnancy, right after the birth, or did it happen later?

    I would have to say once we left the hospital and got home. There were no more nurses, no button to push if I had a question or needed help. We were now on our own and had to figure it out.

6) Did you immediately bond with your baby or did it take a little time? If it did take some time, about how long?

    It took me some time to really bond. My daughter had jaundice and was put back into the hospital to be treated. Then, by week two, she still had jaundice because I did not produce enough milk. She was a very fussy baby and it took us a good month to figure each other out. I feel horrible saying that because now I totally bond with her and have this indescribable love for her. I just adore her and she adores me and that is the coolest thing in the world. I have a purpose now that means more than anything in my past life (prior to kids).

7) Did you find it hard to accept the new responsibilities that a baby brought? Please explain.

    I didn't find it hard to accept the new responsibilities;

they were just new to me. It was a rude awakening that everything that I did in the past was not going to work with this new life. I had to somehow figure out how to function in life with a new baby and that was hard for me.

8) Did you have support (other than a spouse or partner) or seek it out?

I had the support of my husband and family; however, my family lives out of town and my husband works very long hours. By day three I was left alone to figure out this baby and Mom stuff. I had to figure it out, and by week two I went to Mommy and Me because I needed support and I thought I was possibly going crazy.

9) Did having a child change your marriage or your relationship with your partner either positively or negatively? Please explain and/or give examples.

In the beginning it definitely changed my marriage negatively. My life had totally changed and my husband's seemed to continue as business as usual. I really disliked him for that. I didn't feel like he knew what I was going through or like he was even helping me. I clearly had the baby blues and had no clue what I was supposed to do. I was the one getting up in the middle of the night to feed while he slept next to me, snoring.

10) If it did change, were you surprised about this?

I was not surprised by the change. I was warned by other moms that this may happen.

11) Do you work or stay at home?
Work full-time.

12) If you work, how did you cope with the change of going back to work? Was it hard to do? What is it a relief to get back to a routine? What helped you?
I will be returning to work in August.

14) What would you have done differently if you could do it all over again (this answer can cover anything from coming home from the hospital to taking a weekend away to making decisions about your baby)?
I would have asked for more help after the baby was born.

15) Do you find yourself ever feeling like the guilty mommy (for any reason)? If so, how do you cope with this?
I probably feel guilty on a daily basis. Do I hold her too much or not enough? Am I loving her enough...does she know how much I love her...is it okay for her to cry, do I entertain her enough? All of these questions go through my mind on a daily basis.

16) Do you think society portrays a certain image of mothers that we all must aspire to? If so, what is that image and do you think it's possible (or necessary) to become that mom?
I think society really does not let the world know how hard it is to be a mom. We are all supposed to act like it is

this wonderful thing all the time, and the truth is some days I really suck at it and can't stand it, and other days I feel like I am the best mom. I don't think moms want people to know if they are not enjoying being a mom because how dare you even think it. The truth is that it is a hard job and society does not show that.

17) What would be three pieces of advice (practical, inspirational, etc.) that you would give first-time moms?

Really enjoy your old life of picking up at the drop of a hat to go to dinner, shopping, or vacation. Expect the unexpected, know that every baby is different and don't be afraid to try anything. You need to do what works for your baby and try not to listen to negative advice on what you should be doing. In the beginning you are in survival mode and that is okay. The first eight to twelve weeks will be tough, be prepared that it does get better.

18) What is your view of mothers and motherhood today?

I have a newfound respect for my mom as well as any mother that I see in the grocery store or out and about. It is the hardest job but the most rewarding job. The day your child smiles at you it makes all the difference and nothing else really seems to matter.

Any other comments you wish to make?

Being a mom is tough, but I would not change it for the world. Heck, we are already planning when we will start trying for another. :) Hope that helps.

Amy

1) What was your view of mothers and motherhood before you had your own child?

I thought being a mommy would be so fun and always wanted kids. I also thought that pregnancy would be pretty easy and that newborns would just sleep all the time. (Ha ha!)

2) Did you always think you would be a mom, or was the idea of children a changing one?

Yeah, I always wanted to be a mom.

3) What were your first thoughts and feelings after you had your baby?

So amazed at the tiny little person I was holding in my arms! She was so beautiful! I was also VERY overwhelmed and had so many emotions going on at once. It was crazy!

4) Was it hard to believe initially that you were actually a mom? Please explain.

Yes, it is like your life changes overnight! One day you're pregnant and the next day you're responsible for a little life. It was hard to believe that I was really a mom.

5) When did you really start feeling like you were a mother? Was it during pregnancy, right after the birth, or did it happen later?

I remember the first day I really felt like a mom. She was just a few days old and I had been up with her all night. I was listening to a lullaby CD with her, and it hit me that I was a mom and that was something I had always wanted to do. I was amazed at that point how much she meant to me! It was a great moment!

6) Did you immediately bond with your baby or did it take a little time? If it did take some time, about how long?

It took a little time. I would say about a month or so. It was really hard at first because I was in a lot of pain. I had a third-degree tear along with having trouble with breastfeeding. I think it really hindered bonding right away. I knew I loved her, but the bonding took some time.

7) Did you find it hard to accept the new responsibilities that a baby brought? Please explain.

Yes, it was really hard to try to do so much at once while being sleep deprived and also being so sore. I knew that I would have more responsibility, but I really underestimated how much more I would have.

8) Did you have support (other than a spouse or partner) or seek it out?

Yes, I had my husband. At first he was really timid to do anything for her, so I was doing it all on my own. Part of me felt that because I was the mom I should be doing it all. I really wore myself out and eventually realized I really needed his help! Once I started asking him for help and showing him what he needed to do, things got much better!!!

9) Did having a child change your marriage or your relationship with your partner either positively or negatively? Please explain and/or give examples.

Yes, having a child definitely changed our marriage. When she was born, we had just celebrated our one-year wedding anniversary. So we were newlyweds and also just had a baby. We spent a lot less time together and it really strained our marriage in the first year. What I learned is that while a new baby changes so much, it's important not to neglect the relationship. Ours is getting much better now (our little girl is almost two), but it was definitely affected it in the beginning.

10) If it did change, were you surprised about this?

Yes, I was surprised. I didn't think it would be so different. I'm happy, though, that it's getting back on track.

11) Do you work or stay at home?

Work from home.

12) If you work, how did you cope with the change of going back to work? Was it hard to do? What is it a relief to get back to a routine? What helped you?

It was definitely hard going back to work. I work from home so it was definitely a challenge to learn how to work full time and to take care of a baby full time. My mom tried to come visit to help out and my husband helped. I also believe that faith in God helped me the most; it was a really difficult transition.

14) What would you have done differently if you could do it all over again (this answer can cover anything from coming home from the hospital to taking a weekend away to making decisions about your baby)?

I would have planned better financially for maternity leave, since I didn't realize I would make so much less. I would also have researched out more things and tried to give myself a little more "me" time. I really neglected myself and my needs, and I think it affected our lives a lot. I would have also liked to have someone show me (with more patience than the lactation consultants at the hospital) how to nurse my baby.

15) Do you find yourself ever feeling like the guilty mommy (for any reason)? If so, how do you cope with this?

Sometimes I do, especially when it comes to the fact that I didn't get to nurse her for very long. I sometimes feel guilty about that. I try to remind myself of how difficult it was and that hopefully for the next baby I will be more prepared for the challenges. Also, I try to remind myself that I did the best I could.

16) Do you think society portrays a certain image of mothers that we all must aspire to? If so, what is that image and do you think it's possible (or necessary) to become that mom?

In a certain sense, yes. I think moms in society today are portrayed to be supermoms that do everything. I think it's a tough image to live up to. I think it's better to do the best you can and spend as much time with your kids as possible. I think time is the most important thing we can give to our kids.

17) What would be three pieces of advice (practical, inspirational, etc) that you would give first-time moms?

1. Love God with all your heart and he will help you through any situation. 2. Realize that you don't know all the answers and seek advice from other experienced mommies. 3. When things get tough, just remind yourself that you will make it through and enjoy the time you spend with your kids.

18) What is your view of mothers and motherhood today?

Motherhood is a very challenging role, but also VERY wonderful! It's harder than I expected, but I have had so much joy from being a mother, it is great!

Teresa

1) What was your view of mothers and motherhood before you had your own child?

Thinking back, I was never convinced I would have kids. When I was in my teens, and twenties, I viewed marriage and parenthood as very restricting and undesirable. I don't think I began to see the positives of the family unit until I was in my thirties and had met my husband.

2) Did you always think you would be a mom, or was the idea of children a changing one?

See #1.

3) What were your first thoughts and feelings after you had your baby?

I was very concerned about her health and well-being first and foremost. I also remember being in the hospital room a few hours after her birth, and my husband said "hi, sweetheart" and I thought he meant me, but he was talking to the baby. I remember not feeling jealous, but realizing there was a shift and I was no longer the sole focus of his attention, like I always had been.

4) Was it hard to believe initially that you were actually a mom? Please explain.

Yes. I remember thinking "Wow, we're not watching her for somebody else, she is actually ours." I also remember a moment when it really hit me that she was ALWAYS going to be there. It was no longer just the two of us. I was happy about it, but also a little scared and overwhelmed by it.

5) When did you really start feeling like you were a mother? Was it during pregnancy, right after the birth, or did it happen later?

I would say after the birth. Meeting her needs, soothing her, giving her love and comfort, all made me feel like her mom.

6) Did you immediately bond with your baby or did it take a little time? If it did take some time, about how long?

I would say I felt love and concern for her right away, but it took a couple of days to sink in that she was really here and really ours.

7) Did you find it hard to accept the new responsibilities that a baby brought? Please explain.

No, I was accepting of the responsibilities, I just think that it's an exhaustion that you can't fully explain to people. They have to go through it themselves to fully understand. I remember being worried while pregnant when I read that babies needed to eat every two or three hours, and I thought, "I'll never be able to do it. I need my sleep or I'll be a wreck." Sometimes I was a bit of a wreck, but after she was born, I found that it was no longer all about me, but rather all about her. I found that helped make the sleeplessness and constant work more tolerable. But there were times when I just couldn't give anymore, I HAD to sleep. Thankfully, my husband helped a lot.

8) Did you have support (other than a spouse or partner) or seek it out?

We have no family in-state so when my mom's visit after the birth ended, we were on our own. I remember feeling quite isolated. It was nice when I started attending the new moms' support group. Meeting women going through the same struggles and joys helped.

9) Did having a child change your marriage or your relationship with your partner either positively or negatively? Please explain and/or give examples.

It definitely changed our relationship and unfortunately it was for the negative. We struggled more the first year of parenthood in our marriage than we ever had before. We were together six years and married for four before she was born. Being parents brought to light a lot of our differences. We had trouble agreeing on parenting styles and communicating broke down. There are times I wondered if we would make it. Things are better now, but not because we didn't try to work it out. Spending time alone without the baby and nurturing your marriage is crucial, even though it can be hard to do.

10) If it did change, were you surprised about this?
Yes, I was surprised at the conflict my husband and I encountered after becoming parents. We struggled with infertility for three years before we became pregnant with Clare, and ironically that struggle brought us closer together than parenthood did initially.

11) Do you work or stay at home?
Work part-time.

12) If you work, how did you cope with the change of going back to work? Was it hard to do? What is it a relief to get back to a routine? What helped you?
It was hard at first. You always hear about how difficult it is to leave them for the first time, and my experience was no exception. I was comfortable with the daycare I found, but still cried when I walked out the door without

her the first time. Eventually, I was glad to be back to work. I feel the time she spends in daycare benefits her, and I benefit being productive at my job and socializing as well. I feel I have the best of both worlds being able to only work two days a week.

14) What would you have done differently if you could do it all over again (this answer can cover anything from coming home from the hospital to taking a weekend away to making decisions about your baby)?

I kind of regret the moment we first brought her home. It was more tense than I care to remember. My husband was driving me nuts and we were arguing about something, instead of telling baby "welcome home." I don't feel this had any effect on her, but I remember it.

15) Do you find yourself ever feeling like the guilty mommy (for any reason)? If so, how do you cope with this?

Sometimes I feel bad when she cries and I lose my patience with her. I try to learn from my mistakes and do a better job the next time around.

16) Do you think society portrays a certain image of mothers that we all must aspire to? If so, what is that image and do you think it's possible (or necessary) to become that mom?

I think the pressures that mothers put on themselves and on other mothers with views different from their own can be a bit much.

17) What would be three pieces of advice (practical, inspirational, etc.) that you would give first-time moms?

REST! I sometimes see first time moms-to-be out and about, looking like they have a to-do list a mile long and I just want to go up to them and tell them to go home and take a nap. Also, enjoy yourself right now. Indulge yourself with something you enjoy, whether it be a weekday matinee, or a massage, or simply reading a book. Do something you enjoy doing (that being pregnant allows) because your free days are numbered. Lastly, I would say when you read the how-to-deal-with-your-new-baby books, take the advice with a grain of salt. I remember treating the suggestions as gospel and feeling like a failure when it didn't work. You really have to trust yourself and remember that your child will be okay. I can't count the number of times in the beginning I would sweat small things, like the fact that she wasn't on a fixed schedule or she was small for her age. The truth was, genetics and her personality played a bigger role in those things than I did. Enjoy the precious time when they are so young.

18) What is your view of mothers and motherhood today?

I think moms could use to lighten up on themselves a little. It's hard work raising a family today and the pressure we put on ourselves doesn't make it any easier.

Kristen

1) What was your view of mothers and motherhood before you had your own child?

I don't think I really had a view of mothers before I had my own child. Of course we all had our own mothers and knew many others, but I never really paid attention to that role. I was a career woman and was striving to make it in the business world—I didn't really think about being a mother as a career choice.

2) Did you always think you would be a mom, or was the idea of children a changing one?

I always assumed I would have a family, but didn't really think about my role as a mother much.

3) What were your first thoughts and feelings after you had your baby?

I thought it was unbelievable that my husband and I created this new human being and that I already helped nurture him and helped him to grow in my belly for nine months.

4) Was it hard to believe initially that you were actually a mom? Please explain.

I instantly knew I was a mom...of course. That's what we were planning. But trying to wrap my thoughts around what a mom does and all the responsibilities was another story.

5) When did you really start feeling like you were a mother? Was it during pregnancy, right after the birth, or did it happen later?

I didn't really feel like a mom until after my son was

born. Technically, that's when you get the title of mom. Now that I think back, motherhood really starts when your baby is in the womb (albeit it is much easier during pregnancy).

6) Did you immediately bond with your baby or did it take a little time? If it did take some time, about how long?

I feel bonding with your baby is a process. He is like [a] kindred spirit that you have known for a little while, but that you have never seen before. And this new person in your life is very needy and demands all of your time and energy. The love is always there, but it takes a while to recognize the parts of you and your husband wrapped in this new body.

7) Did you find it hard to accept the new responsibilities that a baby brought? Please explain.

I accepted the responsibilities right away— it was our choice to have a baby, but I didn't always know what all the responsibilities entailed, and I didn't always like them or know how to cope with them. The responsibilities are overwhelming for a first-time mother.

8) Did you have support (other than a spouse or partner) or seek it out?

Even though all our relatives live out of town, my mother came to help the first couple of weeks and when I needed help. My spouse has been the biggest support.

9) Did having a child change your marriage or your relationship with your partner either positively or negatively? Please explain and/or give examples.

Of course. Introducing a new permanent member to the family will bring changes. I think we work even better as a team now...just out of necessity. It also gives you a very strong mutual interest and love that transcends any hobby or other reasons you were brought together in the first place.

10) If it did change, were you surprised about this?

I didn't really know what to expect, but the changes were all good and my husband's response to fatherhood has exceeded any of my wildest dreams.

11) Do you work or stay at home?

Stay at home.

13) If you stay at home, are you comfortable with this decision? Do you enjoy being a stay-at-home mom or do you sometimes wish that you had a job to go to. Do you sometimes feel that you should have a job (other than being a mom)?

As a career woman, I always thought I would go back to work within a few months. In fact, it took me about seven to eight months to admit I was a stay-at-home mom. This has been a very difficult career change since my job had been so much a part of how I defined myself and who I was. I didn't think poorly of stay-at-home moms, nor did

I think anything of working moms. I was kind of indifferent to the whole motherhood role since I didn't pay much attention to it before I became one. Just like pregnancy. I never thought about it much, but as soon as I was pregnant, I noticed many more pregnant women on the street.

14) What would you have done differently if you could do it all over again (this answer can cover anything from coming home from the hospital to taking a weekend away to making decisions about your baby)?

Honestly, I'm not sure.

15) Do you find yourself ever feeling like the guilty mommy (for any reason)? If so, how do you cope with this?

Of course...

16) Do you think society portrays a certain image of mothers that we all must aspire to? If so, what is that image and do you think it's possible (or necessary) to become that mom?

Everyone has a different image of what a mom should be like—and that is based upon your own experience with your own mother or those you grew up around.

17) What would be three pieces of advice (practical, inspirational, etc.) that you would give first-time moms?

While you are pregnant, spend more time with your friends who are already moms so you can get a better view into the new life that will be yours soon.

18) What is your view of mothers and motherhood today?

My view of motherhood has totally changed. It is the toughest and most important job in our world. I have so much new wonder and respect for my own mom, having raised two children. I don't know how other moms can make it seem so effortless, knowing how tough it really is.

Tanya

1) What was your view of mothers and motherhood before you had your own child?

I looked at motherhood in a mixed fashion. I thought being a mother was an easy and fun task. But at the same time I felt mothers in general gave up much of their personal time and self for their children.

2) Did you always think you would be a mom, or was the idea of children a changing one?

I never thought about having children until I met my husband almost ten years ago. I thought I would go the career route and did not see a family fitting into the plan.

3) What were your first thoughts and feelings after you had your baby?

I was completely overwhelmed and underprepared. I remember crying on my bed telling my husband that I just could not do this. I suffered from depression after my baby was born and had medical issues related to an emergency C-section. I thought I would never be able to be the mom I wanted to be.

4) Was it hard to believe initially that you were actually a mom? Please explain.

Yes, and sometimes it still is. I never really thought of myself as maternal. When I look at my daughter now, I cannot comprehend the blessing that is in front of me.

5) When did you really start feeling like you were a mother? Was it during pregnancy, right after the birth, or did it happen later?

I did not start feeling like a mom until my daughter was about three months old.

6) Did you immediately bond with your baby or did it take a little time? If it did take some time, about how long?

The first few weeks were very difficult for me. I was going through the motions, but the feelings were not there. I was very depressed. I did not start to bond with my baby until she was about three months old.

7) Did you find it hard to accept the new responsibilities that a baby brought? Please explain.

Frankly, I had no clue how much responsibility and work a baby was going to be. I worked with children, including infants, for the last six years, and even that did not prepare me for what motherhood was really like.

8) Did you have support (other than a spouse or partner) or seek it out?

Yes, although I had a very hard time accepting that I needed it. My sister-in-law and father were a great support. I had either my sister-in-law or father with me for the first six weeks due to my medical condition.

9) Did having a child change your marriage or your relationship with your partner either positively or negatively? Please explain and/or give examples.

Having a baby has brought a great deal of stress to my marriage. My marriage has suffered.

10) If it did change, were you surprised about this?

I was very surprised at the difficulties having a baby brought to my marriage. All of a sudden I felt my husband and I were strangers.

11) Do you work or stay at home?

Stay at home.

13) If you stay at home, are you comfortable with this decision? Do you enjoy being a stay-at-home mom or do you sometimes wish that you had a job to go to. Do you sometimes feel that you should have a job (other than being a mom)?

I knew that I wanted to stay at home with my baby from the start and that has never changed. However, I often wish I had a job to escape to. I feel less worthy just being a stay-at-home mother and often feel that I am looked down at by family and friends.

14) What would you have done differently if you could do it all over again (this answer can cover anything from coming home from the hospital to taking a weekend away to making decisions about your baby)?

First, I would accept help and the fact that I cannot do everything. I would hire out for routine things like shopping and cleaning. I would be honest with myself and my doctor about my emotional health.

15) Do you find yourself ever feeling like the guilty mommy (for any reason)? If so, how do you cope with this?

I feel guilty if I want to take some time for myself. I have had to work very hard at making myself set aside time for me.

16) Do you think society portrays a certain image of mothers that we all must aspire to? If so, what is that image and do you think it's possible (or necessary) to become that mom?

I used to think mothers all had it together. Many of them make it look so easy. I think this is why I was so depressed early on, because I did not have it together and was nothing like what society portrays a mom to be. Now however, I realize how unrealistic society is.

17) What would be three pieces of advice (practical, inspirational, etc.) that you would give first-time moms?

Accept help from anyone who is willing to give it. Learn to count to ten slowly...this too shall pass. There is no right or wrong way. Do what works for you and your baby.

18) What is your view of mothers and motherhood today?
Being a mother is a wonderful blessing. But, society and our own conflicting views often gets in our way of being the best mom we can be. Motherhood is the hardest thing I have ever done, but also the most rewarding.

Any other comments you wish to make?
I thank God every day for my daughter. Being a mom develops a love like no other. I would never have thought I would be so happy to see my daughter healthy and happy.

Leisel

1) What was your view of mothers and motherhood before you had your own child?
Mothers were a boring group of people who had nothing better to do in social situations than sit around and bore people with stories about their children. Motherhood was overrated and made you give up your life for that of your children.

2) Did you always think you would be a mom, or was the idea of children a changing one?
When I was a kid I never wanted kids and never played with dolls. After turning nineteen or so I started wondering about kids but wasn't sure I wanted them. After I got married, my husband and I talked about having kids as a

"someday in the future" kind of event. One day we decided we weren't getting any younger so we better start now!

3) What were your first thoughts and feelings after you had your baby?

I was so worn out I wasn't thinking much beyond "get me out of this bed." Then curiosity about the baby set in, followed closely by terror. I had never been around little kids before, let alone infants, and now I was responsible for this little thing?!!?

4) Was it hard to believe initially that you were actually a mom? Please explain.

Yes. I was really happy to not be pregnant anymore and had not thought much about the next step. Now I had someone dependent on me? I was thirty-two years old and convinced I was still a kid myself, I couldn't have a kid! I still have days, though my son is twenty months old, that I feel like I'm waiting until his parents come back to pick him up!

5) When did you really start feeling like you were a mother? Was it during pregnancy, right after the birth, or did it happen later?

After the birth, after we went home from the hospital (though I did get Mother's Day presents while pregnant!). I started feeling like a mom when I was suddenly on my own taking care of this little scrap of humanity, especially in the middle of the night while my husband slept.

6) Did you immediately bond with your baby or did it take a little time? If it did take some time, about how long?

I got attached pretty quick in the hospital, though not immediately. I was pretty wiped out after birth and not really interested in anything for a while. It was a couple of hours after the birth before they brought my son back to me. Later that day I remember being amazed at how quickly something so new and so small could mean so much to me.

7) Did you find it hard to accept the new responsibilities that a baby brought? Please explain.

Yes! There were days all I wanted to do was take a nap and I couldn't! I still can't handle the smell of baby puke and cleaning up after diaper blow-outs seemed like torture. I got through it and now it seems like less of a big deal, but as a new mom it was really a big deal and I felt very put upon having to do this stuff all the time. My husband got to leave everyday and go to work and talk to grown-ups and I was stuck at home going nuts.

8) Did you have support (other than a spouse or partner) or seek it out?

I had my mom around a little. She was very condescending in her attitude. She liked to say "been there, done that" or "this too shall pass" instead of being actually helpful. When my son was about three months I started going to a Mommy and Me group offered through the hospital I delivered at. My husband actually nagged me until I went to the group a couple of times and started wanting to go for myself.

9) Did having a child change your marriage or your relationship with your partner either positively or negatively? Please explain and/or give examples.

Yes. At first it made things harder in my marriage. My focus shifted completely to baby care and being a mom and I forgot to be much of a wife for a while. It took a while to figure out I had to multitask in that arena too. I got very mad at my husband for a while too because he was going on with life as usual and I had to do "baby duty." His life wasn't seeming to change at all while mine got turned completely upside down. I resented that a lot. Eventually we figured out we needed to talk about the changes and our feelings and we worked through them, but it was rough for a while.

10) If it did change, were you surprised about this?

Honestly, stupid me, I didn't expect our lives to change much at all, we'd just be towing a kid around with us. I was shocked and angry at first about how much our lives and our relationship changed.

11) Do you work or stay at home?
Stay-at-home.

13) If you stay at home, are you comfortable with this

decision? Do you enjoy being a stay-at-home mom or do you sometimes wish that you had a job to go to. Do you sometimes feel that you should have a job (other than being a mom)?

I love being at home with my son. There are days I want to run away screaming but I am glad I am at home with him. Sometimes I feel like I should be contributing financially to our household, but my husband usually reminds me we are saving a huge amount by not having our son in daycare, and I really don't do all that well on the happiness scale having a boss telling me what to do anyway!

14) What would you have done differently if you could do it all over again (this answer can cover anything from coming home from the hospital to taking a weekend away to making decisions about your baby)?

I will not have the huge break in time between having the baby and getting to hold it at the hospital. I think I'll be a bit more relaxed about bringing the next one home, as I now have some experience. Nights out with my husband sooner after the baby is born and more frequently.

15) Do you find yourself ever feeling like the guilty mommy (for any reason)? If so, how do you cope with this?

I feel guilty all the time. It is hard convincing myself it is okay to get a babysitter and go out. I deserve some down time. My child deserves a break from me now and then too. Having a break makes both of us appreciate each other more and strengthens my relationship with my husband. You read that it takes a village to raise a child. I believe that completely... sometimes you have to look hard to find your "village," but find it and let them help. It was also hard for me to convince myself that when people offered help I should take it, it was not an imposition on them... they OFFERED!

16) Do you think society portrays a certain image of mothers that we all must aspire to? If so, what is that image and do you think it's possible (or necessary) to become that mom?

I think society does portray the image of the perfect mom. I don't think it is possible. It's kind of like looking at the models in magazines and realizing "I'm never gonna look like that." I fall more into the category of trying not to give my kid too much to complain about to Oprah when he grows up!

17) What would be three pieces of advice (practical, inspirational, etc.) that you would give first-time moms?

Learn to take a deep breath, a break and/or a nap whenever you can. Those spider webs aren't going anywhere, play with your kid, they grow up too fast and when you blink you miss something. If the diaper really explodes and you just can't deal with it, don't be afraid cut off the outfit and throw it away. Sometimes it just isn't worth washing that out!

18) What is your view of mothers and motherhood today?

Mothers are the most overworked, underappreciated people on the planet! They deserve flowers and candy at least once a week, if not daily!

Kelley

1) What was your view of mothers and motherhood before you had your own child?

It was a bit rose-tinted; I thought mothers, or at least the mom I would become, were the ultimate picture of balance. I didn't base this idea on any one person, but on a collective view of the suburban mom, going to the gym, carting kids to school and practices, making brownie treats, and keeping the house together and being ready for the next meal or potluck...

2) Did you always think you would be a mom, or was the idea of children a changing one?

Always a mom.

3) What were your first thoughts and feelings after you had your baby?

I felt overwhelmed by the gravity of it. I had never been in a role before that was a never-ending, twenty-four hours a day, and that was entirely mine, even with my husband's support. I still feel there's never a real sense of utter relaxation, I mean in the way there was before I had another life to protect.

4) Was it hard to believe initially that you were actually a mom? Please explain.

A little. More in that I couldn't believe I was old enough. I kept recalling families I once babysat for and thought were "older" and realized that's me now.

5) When did you really start feeling like you were a mother? Was it during pregnancy, right after the birth, or did it happen later?

Sometime while I was pregnant, but the feeling still grows as I become more practiced and comfortable with new challenges and milestones.

6) Did you immediately bond with your baby or did it take a little time? If it did take some time, about how long?

No. Not to say I didn't not bond, but I didn't instantly hear music, gaze into her eyes, and feel extraordinary. As her personality developed over the first few months I felt more connected.

7) Did you find it hard to accept the new responsibilities that a baby brought? Please explain.

Yes. Again, motherhood is such a full-time job, from breastfeeding every few hours, to changing, maintaining sleep schedules...I've never been a ultra-scheduled person so I found it difficult to curb my ability to go for a run, dash to the store, or meet up with friends around a baby schedule. I tried and I felt guilty whenever she fussed because I wanted to push the jogger a little farther or find one more thing at the store.

8) Did you have support (other than a spouse or partner) or seek it out?

Some. My parents are nearby and my mom offered to come over every day after work so I could go exercise—as that seemed to be one thing I needed to feel better post-baby body. I realize how fortunate I am to have had that extra time. Really, we chose to live in Nor Cal entirely for the proximity to my family.

9) Did having a child change your marriage or your relationship with your partner either positively or negatively? Please explain and/or give examples.

Both. I think we're striving for a common goal more now and we do agree on parenting skills, which is huge. The most difficult part is a bit of resentment I have for my husband's freedom. He still meets up with friends for lunch, drops by the store or hair salon after work, etc...tasks that for me require an act of Congress. He is very involved and supportive but I feel he'll never understand the full-time nature of motherhood. I think he does manage to relax in a way I never quite accomplish.

10) If it did change, were you surprised about this?
No.

11) Do you work or stay at home?
Work part-time.

12) If you work, how did you cope with the change of going back to work? Was it hard to do? What is it a relief to get back to a routine? What helped you?

My job is unique in that I'm a pediatric nurse at the university hospital. I love exercising my mind, having the social outlet, and experiencing a rewarding career. It's incredibly flexible—I work about two twelve-hour shifts a week as I choose. At first the hard part was returning to a fast paced job and feeling my skills may have slipped. My mom or husband watched my daughter so that was fine. But, that said, my day is so fast and the patients can be so sick that I don't have time to worry about my own child. She's had to go to the ER herself and while my husband called to tell me, I couldn't leave or stop transfusing some other child with blood to rush down and see my own child until I had staff coverage. When I'm at work, I'm committed to being there in a way a lot of other jobs may not require. At the same time, I've found myself emotionally pulling away from some of the horrible situations I encounter, like abuse cases, terminally ill children, and children left alone.

13) If you stay at home, are you comfortable with this decision? Do you enjoy being a stay-at-home mom or do you sometimes wish that you had a job to go to. Do you sometimes feel that you should have a job (other than being a mom)?

I'm at home five days a week—I'm amazed by how much I can get done during a two-hour nap, and yet how little I seem to get done at the same time.

14) What would you have done differently if you could do it all over again (this answer can cover anything from coming home from the hospital to taking a weekend away to making decisions about your baby)?

I would have spent more time connecting with moms in the beginning. I was too fearful my baby was crying too much and people didn't want us around. At the same time I would have stayed home more. I would have written down more milestones.

15) Do you find yourself ever feeling like the guilty mommy (for any reason)? If so, how do you cope with this?

When I'm cleaning or working on some project and I don't get down and play I feel badly. Right now I'm pregnant with #2 and I feel guilty over how tired and sick I've felt. Poor little one has watched so much *Sesame Street* because I was too ill to entertain.

16) Do you think society portrays a certain image of mothers that we all must aspire to? If so, what is that image and do you think it's possible (or necessary) to become that mom?

Yes and no. I don't think it is, although I seem to spot moms around I think are pretty close...or are they? My husband always tries to remind there's always a side you don't see.

17) What would be three pieces of advice (practical, inspirational, etc.) that you would give first time moms?

Always be thankful for what you have. I know that can be relative considering struggles and health issues we all may encounter, but there's always something to appreciate. Rely on others. Don't be afraid to ask for help, because it's surprising how much friends and family will want to help but just don't want to interfere. You don't need to read a zillion books—just go with what seems to make common sense. Do what feels right to you not based on others' comments or rules.

18) What is your view of mothers and motherhood today?
Hardest job ever.

Any other comments you wish to make?
This was surprisingly therapeutic. Thanks.

Recommended Reading and Listening

Books

Daring Greatly: How the Courage to Be Vulnerable Transforms the Way We Live, Love, Parent, and Lead by Brené Brown; Avery; Reprint edition (April 7, 2015)

Good Night, Sleep Tight: The Sleep Lady's Gentle Guide to Helping Your Child Go to Sleep, Stay Asleep, and Wake Up Happy by Kim West; Vanguard Press; (December 22, 2009)

Living What You Want Your Kids to Learn: The Power of Self-Aware Parenting by Cathy Adams; Be U (December 1, 2014)

Podcasts

Zen Parenting Radio—parents Cathy and Todd Adams discuss parenting, life, and how to get the best out of both.

Robcast—Rob Bell is a spiritual leader whose podcast makes us all feel a little better about life.

Happier with Gretchen Rubin—sisters Gretchen and Elizabeth discuss the little ways that we can make our lives happier and the stumbling blocks we often encounter.

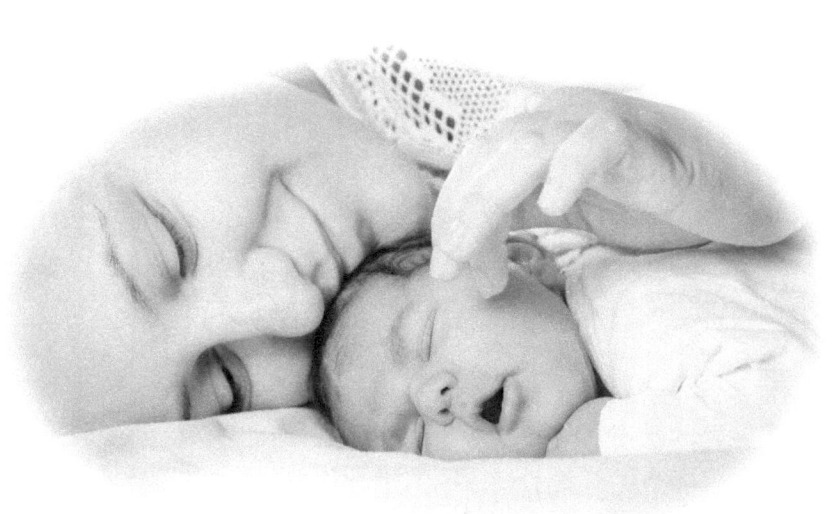

www.ingramcontent.com/pod-product-compliance
Lightning Source LLC
Chambersburg PA
CBHW021146080526
44588CB00008B/245